Praise for
Every Woman's Battle

"This book sheds light on the often unspoken sensitivities and issues that women wrestle with. Not only is it well written, it is liberating and refreshing with sound principles for overcoming the things that threaten to keep us from experiencing the fullness of joy that is part of God's big-picture plan for our lives."

—MICHELLE MCKINNEY HAMMOND, author of *Get Over It and On With It*

"In today's permissive culture, it is dangerously easy for even the most principled of women to reason away unhealthy thoughts, attitudes, and flirtations with men who aren't our husbands. In *Every Woman's Battle,* Shannon Ethridge bravely and respectfully draws a line in the sand for all of us. A must-read for every woman who desires true intimacy and sexual integrity."

—CONSTANCE RHODES, author of *Life Inside the "Thin" Cage*

"There is a common, almost Victorian, myth that women don't really struggle with sexual sin. That myth causes many women to feel a double-shame. The shame of struggling sexually is compounded by the assumption that few, if any, women share the same battle. Shannon Ethridge artfully and boldly unveils the war and offers women a way to enter the battle with courage, hope, and grace. *Every Woman's Battle* will help both men and women comprehend the glorious beauty and sensuality of holiness. This is a desperately needed book."

—Dr. DAN B. ALLENDER, president of Mars Hill Graduate School
and author of *The Healing Path*

"If you're like me, you want the deepest connection possible with your husband. You want a soul-to-soul connection that is not encumbered by anything that could damage it. And if you're like me, you are going to find Shannon's book immeasurably helpful in doing just that. *Every Woman's Battle* is the best resource I know for embracing God's plan of sexual and emotional integrity as a woman."

—LESLIE PARROTT, author of *When Bad Things Happen to Good Marriages*

"A powerful shield for every woman. Shannon's words are convicting, challenging, and confronting."

—Dr. Tim Clinton, president of the American Association
of Christian Counselors

"Many of my *Bad Girls of the Bible* readers have tearfully confessed to me their struggles with sexual sins—promiscuity, adultery, and self-gratification among them. Since we cannot pretend Christian women don't face these temptations, it's a relief to have a sound resource like this one to recommend. Shannon Ethridge's straightforward, nonjudgmental, step-by-step approach can help women come clean in the best way possible—through an intimate relationship with the Lover of their souls."

—Liz Curtis Higgs, best-selling author of *Bad Girls of the Bible,*
Really Bad Girls of the Bible, and *Mad Mary: A Bad Girl from Magdala*

"It's time to take the blinders off and recognize the crucial message of *Every Woman's Battle.*"

—Karen Kingsbury, best-selling author of *Remember* and *One Tuesday Morning*

Readers Rave About
Every Woman's Battle

"Thank you for writing this. I wish I had it when I started dating. I've been a Christian all my life but compromised because I thought I was strong enough. I wondered why I had trouble resisting temptation and kept getting involved with the wrong guy. Now I realize the wrong guys just know what to say. I've read your book twice and will read a couple chapters even more when I feel tempted. I have recommended it to many women." —Shauna

"This weekend, my husband finally realized how his pornography addiction is affecting our marriage. I was full of righteous indignation until your book. I discovered I'm guilty as well. I thank God He used you to help me see my own weaknesses. Now I'm surrendering to Christ for healing and growth." —Lisa

"This book has transformed my relationship with God and my husband. God has worked through you to alter my life and many others, and I can't fully express my gratitude. I feel I've been waiting all my life for this. I finally understand, and my skepticism dissolved at the end of the first page." —ANNE

"I'm thirty-four in Moscow. Your book is great! I started meetings for young girls here, translating off the page, letting them ask questions and make comments. They're very grateful for the book—it's extremely practical and applicable. The things you discuss are so true, but I've never heard anyone mention them. I've attended many women's conferences, but nowhere have I come across such practical, *necessary* information." —RHONDA

"I'm reading your book for the first time and feel beyond blessed! I'm from Puerto Rico, thirty-four years old, and it seems this book is a biography of my life. I still don't believe how timely God's power is in putting this book into my hands. I intend to lead other women in this study so I can share this happiness and freedom with others. I feel so blessed; you have no idea!" —G.F.

"This has long been on my heart, especially being a military wife. Our husbands go out for a year or more at a time, and though we deny it, we struggle with remaining faithful. We pretend we're stronger than we are. I'm facilitating a class for military wives using this book, and I want to thank you for showing us how God provides the way out of temptation." —V.R.

"I've been married for sixteen years, and I know the Lord wanted me to read this book. The timing could not have been better. It's so helpful to know that what I feel is normal. It helps me get over my guilt and get busy (with God's help) dealing with solutions." —B.C.

"This book calls it as it is, and through that, God pointed out issues I needed to think about. It's such a clear guide; I've been reading bits to my boyfriend, helping him understand how women work." —S.B.

"I can't tell you how much reading this has changed my life. Though I'm not 'fixed' yet, I have learned so much and applied it to making our home a happier place. I feel as though you know me inside and out! Your books have played a huge part in saving my marriage. You are doing God's work to change people's lives. *And it's working!*" —L.T.

"All I can say is, 'Wow!' How can God work so profoundly? I was praying about my relational hang-ups, asking how I could love Him while still struggling with these issues. I went to the bookstore the same day and picked up your book. I feel loved, very loved, like someone cares. You helped me receive His unmerited mercy. He really loves us and is a rewarder of those who diligently seek him. I don't know you, but I feel like we've shared in this together." —K.N.

"I just had to tell you I can't even eat my lunch without stopping and thanking you for writing this book, for your honesty and openness about an area so few women talk about. I read my own thoughts that I didn't know anyone else had! I'm experiencing great healing—healing I didn't know was possible." —T.B.

"After stumbling upon your book a few years ago, I can honestly say I've learned more from it than just about any other I've ever read. Thank you, thank you, thank you for writing this incredibly honest and straightforward book—and for changing my life in the process. I cannot say enough. I am reading it again." —ANGELA

"I read your book when I was having an affair and on the verge of losing my husband and family. It was my mirror and the reflection scared me. Reading about your experiences saved my life and my marriage. I've handed out dozens of copies, and now three and a half years later, I'm leading a study with my staff and friends from church. I've seen this book open many women's eyes to their significance and fill the void in their lives. Your passion has touched many lives, and if I have anything to do with it, it will touch many more!" —M.H.

"This is certainly not the last book of yours I'll read. It's opened my eyes! If I had the money, I'd give it to every woman I know!" —AASLAUG, from Norway

SHANNON ETHRIDGE

with Foreword and Afterword by
STEPHEN ARTERBURN

WORKBOOK INCLUDED

Every Woman's Battle

Discovering God's Plan for
Sexual and Emotional Fulfillment

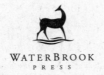

WaterBrook
PRESS

EVERY WOMAN'S BATTLE
PUBLISHED BY WATERBROOK PRESS
12265 Oracle Boulevard, Suite 200
Colorado Springs, CO 80921

Names and facts from stories contained in this book have been changed, but the emotional and sexual struggles portrayed are true stories as related to the author through personal interviews, letters, or e-mails.

ISBN 978-0-307-45798-1

Published in association with the literary agency of Alive Communications Inc., 7680 Goddard Street, Suite 200, Colorado Springs, CO 80920, ww.alivecommunications.com.

Published in the United States by WaterBrook Multnomah, an imprint of the Crown Publishing Group, a division of Random House Inc., New York.

WATERBROOK and its deer colophon are registered trademarks of Random House Inc.

Library of Congress Cataloging-in-Publication Data
Ethridge, Shannon.
  Every woman's battle : discovering God's plan for sexual and emotional fulfillment /
Shannon Ethridge.—1st ed.
    p. cm.
  Includes bibliographical references.
  1. Sex—Religious aspects—Christianity. 2. Love—Religious aspects—Christianity.
3. Women—Religious life. I. Title.
  BT708.E84 2003
  241'.66—dc21

                                              2003005867

Printed in the United States of America
2009

10 9 8 7 6 5 4 3 2

SPECIAL SALES
Most WaterBrook Multnomah books are available at special quantity discounts when purchased in bulk by corporations, organizations, and special-interest groups. Custom imprinting or excerpting can also be done to fit special needs. For information, please e-mail SpecialMarkets@WaterBrookMultnomah.com or call 1-800-603-7051.

To my husband, Greg.
Thank you for your obedience
to God and your faith in me.
Your love has been my strength
and shield in the midst of every battle.

contents

Workbook

foreword

(by Stephen Arterburn)

A couple of years ago, I worked with Fred Stoeker to produce the book *Every Man's Battle*. At first I was reluctant to be involved with the project because I did not think men would want to read a book that so blatantly confronted the battle that almost all men fight, the battle against lust and sexual impurity. So when over four hundred thousand books in the Every Man series sold within two years, it both surprised and encouraged me. I was surprised to see the books remain on the best-seller list and encouraged that men in churches all over the world are addressing an area of their lives that up until now has been a huge secret. A new openness has led to hope for many men who were trapped in their silence and their sins.

Just this morning I was introduced to a young woman named Danielle. She handed me two books that looked like they had been left out in the rain and run over by a garbage truck. The books were *Every Man's Battle* and *Every Woman's Desire*. Danielle explained that they looked so tattered because her husband, David, had read and studied them so much. She told me that David is leading a class of men through the books, and that this is the second time he has done so. I find such dedication to this material and subject matter astounding.

As Danielle and I talked, she told me that her church is taking on a new project. They are using the material from *Every Man's Battle* and creating a group for women to address the same issues. I reached into my briefcase and showed her the manuscript for *Every Woman's Battle*. She was thrilled. But not nearly as much as I was to see her excitement to help other women find the truth her husband and his group of men have found.

Since I helped write *Every Man's Battle,* many women have asked me, "Where is the book to help us with our battle?" In *Every Man's Battle* I gave my e-mail address and asked readers to contact me directly. I have been very busy answering thousands of e-mails from men who are committed to sexual integrity and sexual purity. But men were not the only ones who contacted me. Women read the book and many had the same questions. It was out of those e-mails and face-to-face discussions with women like Danielle that *Every Woman's Battle* emerged.

While it may not be so obvious for women as it is for men, there is a battle that almost every woman will have to fight—the battle for emotional and sexual integrity. But a woman's battle does not usually begin with a lustful or a wandering eye, as it does for a man. While women are visually stimulated as well, their battle is typically more subtle and begins in much deeper territory. For women the battle often begins in a heart full of disappointment.

A woman's disappointment in men, circumstances, God, life, money, kids, and the future can cause her heart to wander. If she's single she may turn to fantasy and self-gratification, hurting her potential to develop a healthy sexual connection with her future husband. If she's married, she may start comparing her husband with every other man, and when she does, he always comes up short. She may obsess over all that he is not and all that he could be. She may express her desires for him to be different and better, creating criticisms and complaints in almost every conversation. It becomes so serious that she begins to feel entitled to something better, someone who can meet her needs the way she deserves. Unknowingly she betrays her husband with almost every thought of him and someone else she views as superior. And with each comparison comes a greater and deeper disconnection between the two of them and the increasing likelihood that she may fall into an emotional affair or even a sexual one. But even if she does neither, her rejection of her husband destroys the potential for her to experience the fulfillment she longs for.

I believe that women want a deep connection with a man—a connection that is so deep it grows into an inseparable intimacy that results in great satisfaction as friends as well as sexual partners. But in order for this to happen, men and women have to live lives of sexual integrity. For men, that means keeping our minds and hearts from other women, including pornographic images and sexual memories from the past. For women, that means accepting rather than rejecting their husbands. It means overcoming disappointment to keep their connection with their husbands healthy.

When I heard Shannon's story and met her, I knew she could write this book.

She has experienced the temptations that most women are too embarrassed or afraid to admit. For years she had a wandering heart—but no longer. Shannon's heart was healed as she embraced God's plan for sexual and emotional fulfillment. Her openness, wisdom, honesty, and integrity can help you live a life of sexual and emotional integrity as well.

In order for you to grow and mature, your sexuality must be integrated into the rest of your life. That means integrating your thought life and fantasy life into your marriage. When you do, you feel complete, congruent, and whole. The danger of living in your private world of fantasy and gratification is that you end up with a segmented life, one with secret fantasies, secret sexual practices, and obsessions. If this describes you, this book will show you how to integrate all parts of your being so that you become a whole and healthy woman, faithfully connected in intimacy with your mate and your God.

If you have been wandering in the disappointing world of what was and what might have been, *Every Woman's Battle* will bring you back to the reality of what God wants you to be and what your marriage can be. Married or single, you can find help and hope within these pages. I pray that when you are finished reading you will be on a path of spiritual growth and maturity that will allow you to stand pure before the Lord and experience true sexual and emotional fulfillment.

May God bless you greatly for your desire to seek His truth.

P.S. This book was written primarily for women who are married or plan to be. If you are single, this book will be invaluable as you are envisioning a fulfilling marriage. If you are not planning on being married, it will help you give wise counsel to your friends.

acknowledgments

My deepest gratitude goes first to Jesus Christ, the Lover I've longed for all my life. Thank You for revealing Yourself to me and for trusting me with Your vision for Well Women Ministries. Thank You also for the precious gift of a godly husband. Greg, where would I be had you not loved me as Christ loved the church, especially in the midst of my most "unlovable" moments? Your example of faithfulness through the past thirteen years has proven that true, unconditional love isn't just a fairy tale. No writer could compose words deep enough to express my love and commitment to you.

Thank you to my children, Erin and Matthew, for believing in me and cheering me on. The sunshine and laughter you bring into each day is such a gift. Of all the hats I wear in life, I'm most proud of my "Supermom" hat. You are incredible kids!

To Mom and Pop—oh, how I appreciate your discipline, patience, and prayers. I was very lucky to have you as parents, more lucky now to have you as friends. To Jay and Wanda—thank you for loving me like a daughter and for raising such a great son. What a joy to have parents and parents-in-law who are so supportive.

Thank you to all my "other mothers" in the Little Flock Sunday-school class for praying me through the peaks and valleys in life. What an example you have set for me.

To my accountability friends who helped me see the Light when I was blinded by Satan's schemes. Lisa, whoever said blood is thicker than water didn't know about the fierce friendship that we share! I love you so much.

To Ron and Katie Luce, David Hasz, and all my colaborers in Christ at Teen Mania Ministries. Your encouragement, inspiration, and trust is so much of what God used to keep me pressing on with this manuscript and ministry. It is an honor and a privilege to work with you to raise up a generation of Worldchangers! To

Kym Blackstock and Tracy Kartes, you came alongside me at such a vital time in this writing process, and I am grateful for your assistance.

To Jack Hill, Dean Sherman, and all of our friends at Mercy Ships International, with sincere appreciation for the wisdom gleaned and the hope and healing you allow us to spread to women in other parts of the world.

To my phenomenal mentors, Jerry Speight and Susan Duke—you have been wind underneath my wings! Jerry, you have encouraged me to pursue avenues that I never dreamed of walking down. Thank you for inspiring me to become all God intended. And Susan, my "hen with a pen" friend—thank you for adopting this baby chick and giving me "eggstra" courage to press on!

Special thanks to all those who came alongside me to get this project into the hands of many other women. Linda Glasford and Greg Johnson, thank you for catching this vision and taking a chance on me. All of the pink roses and seashells in the world wouldn't express the magnitude of my appreciation. Stephen Arterburn and Fred Stoeker, thank you for sharing my passion for starting a new kind of revolution! What a privilege to be invited to come alongside you in this movement. Finally, to my incredible editor, Liz Heaney, and to all the wonderful folks at WaterBrook Press, a sincere thank you for your patience and professionalism in helping me develop this manuscript into something that I pray will be instrumental in changing many lives.

One day my husband, Greg, brought home the book *Every Man's Battle,* tossed it at me, and with a straight face said, "I think you ought to write *Every Woman's Battle.*"

My immediate response was, "Yeah, right!" Not that I didn't feel qualified to write such a book (having graduated from the school of hard knocks when it comes to recognizing and overcoming sexual and emotional temptations), but I had already been trying to publish a manuscript on these exact issues for over a year. Time after time I heard publishers say, "Women don't deal with sexual issues enough that a book on that topic would really sell."

Meanwhile, *Every Man's Battle* was climbing to the top of the best-seller list. I wondered how people could be so naive as to think that sexual integrity is strictly a man's issue. Both men and women were created by God as sexual beings, weren't they? It takes two to tango, and for every man who falls prey to sexual temptation, there is a woman falling with him. While many men limit their affairs to what they take in lustfully through their eyes, women also submit longingly to mental fantasies or emotional affairs. Some compare their husbands to other men and become disillusioned by their husbands' failure to measure up. So many of us fail to recognize how we compromise our sexual integrity, how we rob ourselves of what we long for most—true intimacy and fulfillment.

Curious as to why my husband felt so strongly about *Every Man's Battle,* I read it through voraciously. I kept thinking, *Many of these issues are not common just to men, but to women also! They simply manifest themselves differently!*

Stephen Arterburn was hearing the exact same thing from so many women that he believed the need was undeniable. Little did I know that within a few months God would, in fact, divinely bring Steve and me together on this project (thanks to my friends Ron and Katie Luce, our literary agents at Alive Communications, and the visionaries at WaterBrook Press).

So take heart and know that your cries for help have been heard. This book is a training manual that will help you avoid sexual and emotional compromise and will show you how to experience God's plan for sexual and emotional fulfillment. I also wrote a comprehensive workbook to accompany *Every Woman's Battle*. It will help you learn more about what God has to say on this subject and will help you examine your own personal life so you can develop a practical plan for victory in your own unique battle for sexual and emotional integrity.

Do you want to be a woman of sexual and emotional integrity? With God's help you can. Let's get started.

PART I

understanding
where we are

not just a man's battle!

You stumble day and night....
My people are destroyed from lack of knowledge.

HOSEA 4:5-6

At one time I was having extramarital affairs with five different men.

First, there was Scott. I met him while volunteering at a summer camp. Scott was so outgoing and talkative. What initially attracted me to him was how he could have a conversation with anyone—not just a superficial one, but a deep, meaningful discussion. I could walk into a room and he would pour on the attention, asking all about how things were going and how I was feeling. In comparison, however, my husband was a man of few words: the strong, silent type.

Then there was my scuba coach, Mark. With his distinguished, salt-and-pepper hair, he looked just like Lloyd Bridges. Mark's maturity and love for diving intrigued me. He encouraged me to overcome my fears and helped me discover my underwater adventuresome side. I felt safe with him, like a daughter feels safe with her dad. My husband, on the other hand, was only a few years older than I. He didn't evoke within me a feeling of being nurtured and safe as Mark did.

Tom was my accounting teacher at the university I attended. What struck me about Tom was his wit and intelligence. I had expected accounting to be the most boring of all my classes, but Tom had a way of making it the most fun and interesting part of my day. My husband was an intelligent accountant also, but he couldn't make me laugh like Tom did. His wit paled in comparison to Tom's.

Then there was Ray. He had been my boyfriend before I married Greg. Ray was such a die-hard romantic, heaping compliments on me and sweeping me off my feet with whirlwind passion. My relationship with my husband never seemed to have that magic spark that I felt when I was with Ray. Ray had set the romantic standard that my husband couldn't live up to.

Finally, there was Clark. He was ruggedly handsome, suave, and debonair. I looked forward to being with him every Friday night. As I approached the counter at the movie rental store, the owner automatically went to the Classics section and pulled out any Clark Gable movie. It didn't matter which one. I loved them all. Even standing tall at six foot and seven inches, my husband just couldn't measure up to Clark.

Even though I wasn't having sexual intercourse with any of these other men, I was still having an affair with each of them—a mental and/or emotional affair. My fantasies of being Clark Gable's leading lady, memories of my romantic relationship with Ray, and fascination with Tom's wit, Mark's maturity, and Scott's verbal talents affected my marriage in a way just as damaging as a sexual affair would have.

I was overlooking all of the many wonderful things about my husband because I was either focusing on the positive attributes of one of these other men or focusing on my husband's negative attributes. Because I lived with Greg, I saw not just the good, but also the bad and the ugly. He left the toilet seat up in the middle of the night. He snored, and when he woke up he had morning breath. Then he'd brush his teeth and leave toothpaste in the sink. Sometimes I felt that Greg couldn't do anything to suit me. With all of my criticizing, he probably felt like he couldn't do anything to suit me, either.

The other men's warts, however, were out of my line of sight. I could look at them and see nothing but their shining qualities, the kind I initially saw in Greg but had lost sight of over the years because of all my comparisons.

I felt distanced and disillusioned. Could he ever excite me like the other men did? Was I still in love with him? Could he ever measure up? Could I ever learn to live with my less-than-perfect partner?

Fortunately, the positive answers to these questions have surfaced since I ended these affairs and changed my measuring stick. I am thrilled to report that our marriage of thirteen years is still going strong and has never been better (although we, like any other couple, still have our moments). I'm thankful I never traded Greg in for another model and even more thankful that he didn't give up on me, either.

Together, we have discovered a new level of intimacy that we didn't know existed, all because I stopped comparing and criticizing and began embracing the uniqueness of my spouse.

Over the past decade of pursuing my own healing from these (and other) issues, as well as teaching on the topic of sexual purity and restoration, I have come to understand that in some way or another sexual and emotional integrity is a battle that every woman fights. However, many women are fighting this battle with their eyes closed because they don't believe they are even engaged in the battle. Many believe that just because they are not involved in a physical, sexual affair they don't have a problem with sexual and emotional integrity. As a result, they engage in thoughts and behaviors that compromise their integrity and rob them of true sexual and emotional fulfillment.

Let me show you what I mean by introducing you to a few women whose eyes are closed to the compromises they are making.

Rebecca has been happily married for over ten years and says that her husband is very sensitive and caring in bed.

> Craig has always been as concerned with my sexual pleasure as he is with his own. I feel as if it is important to him that I have an orgasm, so most of the time when we are making love, I just close my eyes and imagine being with another man. It's not a man that I know or anything. It's just an imaginary face and body who excites me because I don't know him and it feels dangerous, you know? The thought of being seduced by this stranger in some exotic place puts me in the mood for sex. I can't seem to get into that mood just sitting around the house with my husband. It's not that he's not attractive; I just get more excited at the thought of a dangerous liaison with someone whose socks I don't have to pick up off of the floor.
>
> I would never actually do such a thing (at least I don't think I would), it's just that I feel obligated to climax, and fantasizing about another man just seems to be the only way I can do that. I don't think there's anything wrong

with it, but I joked about it with Craig one day and now he is making a big deal out of it. He says he feels betrayed that I am not 'mentally present' with him during our lovemaking. He says there is no difference between what I am doing and his looking at pornography, but I don't agree. There's nothing wrong with this if I'd never really be unfaithful to him, is there? Doesn't every woman do this?

Carol is a very attractive woman in her midforties and has been married for over twenty years. She and her husband, Chris, are leaders in their church and serve as "marriage mentors" to couples in the congregation needing help in their relationship. However, Chris often travels out of town with his job, and Carol is left to fly solo with some sticky counseling situations.

Several months ago Carol received a call around 9 P.M. from Steve, a longtime member of her Sunday-school class. It was public knowledge that Steve's wife had been an alcoholic for many years, and on this particular night her drunken rampage had sent Steve running for cover. He asked Carol if he could come over and talk with her and Chris for a little while.

"I knew better than to invite Steve to the house since Chris wasn't home. After all, he was very vulnerable—and very handsome. I suggested we meet for coffee at a local deli instead. His anguish really tugged on my heartstrings. We talked past midnight, and I suggested we pray together and then head home since the deli was trying to close up."

As Carol bowed her head with her hands clasped on the tabletop, she felt Steve's strong hands envelop hers and she listened as he poured out his heart in prayer. "Lord, help my wife to see what she could be if she would just sober up. Help her to be more patient and kind and caring…like Carol."

Months later, Carol still spends time imagining becoming even more intimate with Steve. As a matter of fact, things between her and Chris have gotten tense, as Carol often becomes angry or depressed for no apparent reason. "It just seems like every time I hear Steve speak in Sunday school, I hang on to every word and wonder what else I can do to ease his pain without causing any suspicion that I have developed strong feelings for him. Some days I tell myself that I need to confess this to Chris and to our pastor and remove myself from the marriage mentoring program for a while. However, there are many other days that I think, *I'm not doing anything to compromise my marriage, so stop feeling guilty! Just because I find Steve attractive doesn't mean that I shouldn't try to help him.*

Twenty-eight and single, Sandra has been masturbating often for over fifteen years. Her struggle began at age twelve, when she found one of her mother's Harlequin romance novels. A voracious reader, Sandra was soon devouring several novels per week, becoming sexually aroused and often masturbating to get "relief." Sandra confesses:

> By the time I was out of high school, I was regularly holding a book in one hand and stimulating myself with the other. While I felt in my heart that what I was doing was wrong, I could always justify it. After all, the Bible did not expressly forbid it. God had made my body to be responsive, so He surely wouldn't deny me this pleasure, would He? Since He had not given me a husband, I felt it was my right. Surely He couldn't expect me to wait that long, could He? And who was I hurting? No one else was involved.
>
> However, I have always felt as if there is this barrier between me and God. I have sensed Him calling me to stop this behavior, to turn away from it, but the desire is so strong. I stopped reading the romance novels several years ago, but I still fantasize when I am lying in bed by myself, and I usually end up masturbating. I always say to myself, "I'll be obedient tomorrow or next week, but for right now, I just need the release." Sometimes I even get angry with God and think, *If you would give me a husband, I wouldn't have this problem!*

Lacy has been married seven years and has two young children. Even though she and her husband, David, got along great while they were dating, things have steadily gone south in their marriage because of financial pressures. Since David got laid off last year, he's had to do odd jobs to make ends meet. He took one job throwing a paper route in a neighborhood across town. He gets up at 4 A.M. to take care of the paper route responsibilities and then goes to whatever job the temporary agency has for him that day. Lacy complains:

> All David wants to do is work, come home to eat, and then go straight to bed. He shows little interest in spending time with me or helping out with the kids. It's a good thing that we don't want any more children because we rarely ever have sex anymore.
>
> I get jealous when I see other husbands grocery shopping with their wives, going to church with their families, taking their kids to the park, and stuff like that. I confessed this to a friend one day, and she said that the grass is always greener on the other side of the fence. She preached me a little sermon about coveting thy neighbor's husband, so I just shut up.
>
> Even though I would never divorce because I take my wedding vows seriously, I often wonder if David will die before me so that maybe I can have the chance at a happier marriage with a more successful and attentive husband someday. I often dream about that, usually as I lie in bed by myself in the morning after David has already left for his paper route. Somewhere between being fully awake and fully asleep, I have dreams about going on a date with a new guy who wants to take us all out to eat or about a new husband who is in the kitchen preparing to bring me breakfast in bed.

SEEDS OF COMPROMISE, HARVESTS OF DESTRUCTION

Even though none of these women could be tried in a court of law for marital unfaithfulness and convicted of adultery, haven't they been sowing seeds of compromise? Doesn't emotional and mental unfaithfulness still compromise our sexual integrity?

Scripture warns about this very thing:

The one who sows to please [her] sinful nature, from that nature will reap destruction. (Galatians 6:8)

But each one is tempted when, by [her] own evil desire, [she] is dragged away and enticed. Then, after desire has conceived, it gives birth to sin; and sin, when it is full-grown, gives birth to death. (James 1:14-15)

In these scriptures we are called to righteous living. This is the principle: The pursuit of fleshly desires will end in our ultimate demise. When we sow emotional and mental seeds of compromise, we reap a harvest of relational destruction. Just ask Jean.

CAUGHT IN THE WEB OF INTRIGUE

Jean is in her late thirties and married to Kevin, a computer salesman. Once all of their children entered school, Jean decided to reconnect with some old friends during her extra free time. With the first big telephone bill, Kevin insisted that Jean learn to use e-mail to cut down on the expense of all this "reconnecting" she was doing! Being the adept computer salesman that he was, Kevin convinced Jean that she could learn to use the Internet just like everyone else.

She loved this new hobby of forwarding cute e-mails, surfing the Web for coupons, bidding for antiques on eBay, scanning and sending pictures in cyberspace, and so on. Then Jean discovered chat rooms.

A few minutes in a chat room each day grew into several hours each day. One morning while waiting for her buddies to log on, she read a question from someone with the screen name of MiamiMike. "Is *anyone* out there yet or am I in this room alone?"

After a few moments, Jean responded, "Looks like it's just you and me!" By the time Jean's friends finally entered the chat room half an hour later, she and Mike had found out quite a bit about each other—quite a bit they had in common, in fact. Jean grew up in Florida and absolutely loved the beach. Reading about Mike's oceanfront condo while sitting in her snowy Minnesota home gave her cabin fever.

Jean began dropping the kids off at school and heading straight back home to go online, knowing that Mike would be expecting her. Once Mike asked her to log back on that evening so they could chat again before he went to bed. That night, Jean tucked the children in bed, lay down with Kevin until he fell asleep, then tiptoed out of their bedroom and into the study where MiamiMike was waiting. Jean felt deceitful, but thought, *After all, he's hundreds of miles away! What could possibly happen with that much distance separating us?*

The emotional bond between Jean and MiamiMike grew as thick as wet cement. Several weeks later, curiosity got the best of Jean, and she asked Kevin if she could fly back to Florida for the weekend to reunite with some old school girlfriends. "Sure, honey. I can manage," Kevin responded, thinking he had done her a favor. He had actually just given Jean enough rope to hang herself.

Within seventy-two hours, she was on a plane bound for Miami. Pleasantly surprised, MiamiMike met Jean at the airport and escorted her to his condo where a chilled bottle of champagne and two stems of crystal were waiting beside the hot tub. (We'll hear from Jean later in the book.)

NOT JUST A MAN'S BATTLE!

Jesus said:

> You have heard that it was said, "Do not commit adultery." But I tell you
> that anyone who looks at a woman lustfully has already committed adultery
> with her in his heart. (Matthew 5:27-28)

Was He speaking strictly to men here? Absolutely not! To help us apply this scripture to our own lives, let's paraphrase the verse this way:

> I tell you that any woman who envisions a man longingly has already committed adultery with him in her heart.

When I hear people say that women don't struggle with sexual issues like men do, I cannot help but wonder what planet they are from or what rock they have been hiding under. Perhaps what they really mean is, the *physical* act of sex isn't an overwhelming temptation for women like it is for men.

Men and women struggle in different ways when it comes to sexual integrity. While a man's battle begins with what he takes in through his eyes, a woman's begins with her heart and her thoughts. A man must guard his eyes to maintain sexual integrity, but because God made women to be emotionally and mentally stimulated, we must closely guard our hearts and minds as well as our bodies if we want to experience God's plan for sexual and emotional fulfillment. A woman's battle is for sexual *and* emotional integrity.

While a man needs mental, emotional, and spiritual connection, his physical needs tend to be in the driver's seat and his other needs ride along in the back. The reverse is true for women. If there is one particular need that drives us, it is certainly our emotional needs. That's why it's said that men *give love to get sex* and women *give sex to get love*. This isn't intended to be a bashing statement, it's simply the way God made us.

Another unique difference between men and women is that many men are capable of giving their bodies to a partner without feeling the need to give their mind, heart, or soul, whereas women are relatively unable to do this. He can enjoy the act of sex without committing his heart or bonding spiritually with the object of his physical desire. A woman's body, however, goes only to someone whom she

MEN	WOMEN
• crave physical intimacy	• crave emotional intimacy
• give love to get sex	• give sex to get love
• body can disconnect from mind, heart, and soul	• body, mind, heart, and soul intricately connected
• stimulated by what they see	• stimulated by what they hear
• recurrent physical needs cycle	• recurrent emotional needs cycle
• vulnerable to unfaithfulness in the absence of physical touch	• vulnerable to unfaithfulness in the absence of emotional connection

Figure 1.1

thinks of night and day and with whom her heart and spirit have already connected (unless there is dysfunctional or addictive behavior involved). When she gives her mind, heart, and soul, her body is usually right behind. The four are intricately connected (more about this in the next chapter).

While men are primarily aroused by what they see with their eyes, women are more aroused by what they hear. He may fantasize about watching a woman undress, but she fantasizes about him whispering sweet nothings in her ear. The temptation to look at pornography can be overwhelming to a male, while females would much rather read the relational dialogue in a romance novel. Men want to look and touch, whereas women much prefer to talk and relate.

Most men experience a regular, recurring need for a physical, sexual release. Some feel this intense need as often as every couple of days. Others experience it a couple of times per week or even less (according to their season of life). While the frequency of the need varies from man to man, each one has his own sexual "cycle" in which he experiences these physical desires. While it may be difficult for some women to fathom that sex is actually a cyclical need for men, don't we have our own unique cycle as well? Although physical pleasure may not be a cyclical need, we long for attention and affection on a regular, recurring basis.

Just as a man would become far more vulnerable to a sexual affair if his wife rarely responded to his physical needs for a sexual release, a woman becomes far more vulnerable to an affair when her emotional needs are neglected over and over. When a woman falls into a sexual affair, most often her affair begins as an emotional one. It is out of her emotional needs that her heart cries out for someone to satisfy her innermost desires to be loved, needed, valued, and cherished. A woman's emotional needs are just as vitally important to her as a man's physical needs are to him.

Figure 1.1 (on the previous page) summarizes the distinguishing differences between how men and women respond sexually.

NAIVETÉ IS NOT A VIRTUE

Let's not be naive enough to believe that because Rebecca, Carol, Sandra, or Lacy are not acting out physically with a premarital or extramarital partner that their actions aren't compromising their sexual integrity. Nor is it wise to think that what happened to Jean or any of the other women could never happen to us.

The apostle Paul writes:

So, if you think you are standing firm, be careful that you don't fall!... Therefore, prepare your minds for action; be self-controlled.... Do not conform to the evil desires you had when you lived in ignorance. But just as he who called you is holy, so be holy in all you do; for it is written: "Be holy, because I am holy."... Among you there must not be even a hint of sexual immorality. (1 Corinthians 10:12; 1 Peter 1:13-16; Ephesians 5:3)

Paul understood our very human tendency to live in denial, closing our eyes to the things in our lives that may need to change. Change is hard work, and we would rather stay as we are. But this is not how God has called us to live. He wants to help us control our minds and our desires so that we can be more like Him. He wants to help us discover His plan for relational satisfaction. But we can't do this if we insist on keeping our eyes closed to the compromise that robs us of ultimate sexual and emotional fulfillment.

To help you open your eyes to your own struggle for sexual and emotional integrity, I encourage you to take the following quiz.

ARE YOU ENGAGED IN A BATTLE?

Please put a checkmark in the Yes or No column in response to the following questions:

Yes/No

1. Is having a man in your life or finding a husband something that dominates your thoughts? _____

2. If you have a man in your life, do you compare him to other men (physically, mentally, emotionally, or spiritually)? _____

3. Do you often think of what your life will be like after your husband is dead, wondering who the "next man" in your life could be? _____

4. Do you have sexual secrets that you don't want anyone else
   to know about? _____

5. Do you feel like a nobody if you don't have a love interest
   in your life? Does a romantic relationship give you a sense
   of identity? _____

6. Do you seem to attract bad or dysfunctional relationships
   with men? _____

7. Do men accuse you of being manipulative or controlling? _____

8. Do you feel secretly excited or powerful when you sense that
   a man finds you attractive? _____

9. Do you have a difficult time responding to your husband's
   sexual advances because you feel he should meet your needs
   first? _____

10. Is remaining emotionally or physically faithful to one person
    a challenge for you? _____

11. Do you often choose your attire in the morning based on the
    men you will encounter that day? _____

12. Do you find yourself flirting or using sexual innuendos (even
    if you do not intend to) when conversing with someone you
    find attractive? _____

13. Do you resent the fact that your husband wants sex more often
    than you do, or wish that he would just masturbate so that you
    would not have to perform sexually? _____

14. Do you have to masturbate when you get sexually aroused? _____

15. Do you read romance novels because of the fantasies
    they evoke within you or because they arouse you
    sexually? _____

16. Have you ever used premarital or extramarital relationships
    to "medicate" your emotional pain? _____

17. Is there any area of your sexuality that (1) is not known by
    your husband, (2) is not approved of by your husband, or
    (3) does not involve your husband? _____

18. Do you spend more time or energy ministering to the needs of others through church or social activities than to your husband's sexual needs? _____

19. Do you use pornography either alone or with a partner? _____

20. Do you fantasize about being intimate with someone other than your husband? _____

21. Do you have a problem making and maintaining close female friends? _____

22. Do you converse with strangers in Internet chat rooms? _____

23. Have you ever been unable to concentrate on work, school, or the affairs of your household because of thoughts or feelings you are having about someone else? _____

24. Do you think the word *victim* describes you? _____

25. Do you avoid sex in your marriage because of the spiritual guilt or dirty feeling you experience afterward? _____

There is no "magic number" that will determine your level of sexual or emotional integrity. However, if reading through these questions has awakened you to the fact that your sexual activity, romantic behavior, or emotional attachments are a hindrance to your spiritual growth or intimacy in marriage, this book is designed to help you achieve victory in your area of struggle.[1]

Let's open our eyes to understand this gift of sexuality more fully and to dispel some of the myths that have perhaps kept you, like many other women, entrenched in this battle. The coming chapters will help you to:

1. understand the complexity of sexuality and better understand women's unique struggle with emotional integrity (chapter 2);

2. recognize the myths about sexuality that dominate our culture and how they affect a woman's sexual integrity (chapters 3 and 4);

3. control your tendencies to look for love in all the wrong places, whether this is a physical, mental, or emotional battle for you (chapters 5-8);

4. reconnect with your husband (or connect with your future husband) so that you can enjoy the sexual and emotional fulfillment God intends for marriage (chapter 10); and

5. avoid placing unrealistic expectations on your current or future husband and connect with the only true source of fulfillment (chapter 11).

If you have wondered why you feel so disconnected from God, your spouse, or others, this book could be your answer. My prayer is that within these pages you will find hope, healing, and restoration.

a new look
at sexual integrity

I, the LORD, have called you in righteousness;
>   I will take hold of your hand.
I will keep you and will make you
>   to be a covenant for the people
>   and a light for the Gentiles,
to open eyes that are blind,
>   to free captives from prison
>   and to release from the dungeon those who sit in darkness.

ISAIAH 42:6-7

Janet, in her midthirties, has had numerous lunch meetings over the past few years with her good friend Dave, a coworker in an architectural firm. Dave is married, but he doesn't talk much about his wife, which leads Janet to wonder if his marriage will last. Dave and Janet's boss asked their work team to participate in a continuing education conference in Minneapolis, but when Janet realized that they were the only two members of the group who were able to attend the conference, she began stepping through an emotional minefield. Janet confesses:

> I keep imagining Dave and me sitting next to each other on the plane, stirring each other intellectually like our conversations always do. I imagine his hotel room being right down the hall from mine and how he might walk me

to my door and decide to come in so we can continue our conversation. We talk until all hours of the night, and then when he hugs me good-bye like he always does, I feel his body hesitate as he tries to pull away. If he is as attracted to me as I am to him, my fear (or hope) is that this is what will really happen. If he gets weak, I'm almost sure I'll succumb to whatever he wants to do. I know I probably shouldn't go on this trip at all with these ideas in my head, but I can't imagine not going, either.

Has Janet crossed the line when it comes to sexual integrity?

Kelly's secret has been eating her alive for over ten years:

As a freshman in college, I began dating Sam, an older man who was far more sexually experienced than I was. I fell head over heels in love with him, and within a few months, we were sleeping together. Within a year, we were living together. That was when I stumbled upon his vast array of videos hidden on the top shelf of his closet. I'm embarrassed to say that at the time, I wasn't offended by his pornography collection, but curious. I began watching the videos with him, just to see what was on them. It wasn't long until I was asking to watch particular ones while we were having sex together. I don't understand why, but the ones that really turned me on were the ones that included a threesome (a guy and two girls) or the ones that had just two women together.

Even after Sam and I broke up, I asked him if I could keep the couple of videos that were my favorites. I masturbated to them over and over, but when I got married to a Christian man who I knew wouldn't approve of them, I threw them away. That's been years ago, but I've never been able to get these images out of my mind. Even though my husband is a good lover, I think about all those old scenes when I'm trying to orgasm just because that is what really seems to do it for me. I would never actually want to be with a woman in real life, so I don't understand why these fantasies are such a big part of my sex life. I'm afraid if my husband knew about them, he'd think he married a lesbian.

Has Kelly crossed the line when it comes to sexual integrity?

In her midforties, Caroline confesses that her biggest battle in life has been not to compare herself to others. In the women's locker room, Caroline finds herself comparing the size of her waist and hips, the firmness of her breasts, and the amount of "cottage cheese" in her thighs with each passerby. "If I am changing clothes in the presence of a larger woman, I feel lean and powerfully pretty. But let a skinny-minny walk in, and I do a double take at the image staring back at me in the mirror and think, *Yuck!*"

Unfortunately this comparison trap not only affects Caroline's self-esteem, but has carried over into her marriage of sixteen years as well. Although she describes their relationship as "okay," Caroline also admits:

Sometimes I just wish Wendel could be more like some of our friends. I love the way Bill can always make me laugh; Wendel wouldn't know a joke if it bit him. Bob is so handy with tools and builds all kinds of neat things for their house; Wendel couldn't build a birdhouse if his life depended on it. Larry is so attentive to his wife, always bringing her flowers or taking her on getaway weekends; Wendel's idea of a date is sitting in the same room to watch *Wheel of Fortune* together. If he were a little more entertaining to be with, I might feel more like being intimate with him, but it's hard to get excited when this is as good as it gets.

Has Caroline crossed the line of sexual integrity?

Many would say that Janet, Kelly, and Caroline have not yet crossed the sexual integrity line simply because they have stopped short of sexual intercourse outside of marriage. But I disagree; they have each crossed the line by compromising in specific ways. To help you better understand what sexual and emotional integrity look like for a woman, let's talk about "tabletop sexuality."

TABLETOP SEXUALITY: BALANCE AND INTEGRITY

When I address tabletop sexuality in seminars, some people blush, assuming I am referring to the variety of sexual positions or places in the house that a couple can experiment with. Don't panic. Tabletop sexuality is a word picture I use to help women better understand the meaning of sexual integrity. Just as a table has four legs that support it, four distinct components comprise our sexuality. If one of the legs is missing or broken, the table is out of balance, and it becomes a slide.

Some friends of mine discovered this concept at their wedding reception. Following the ceremony, Kevin and Ruth proceeded to the reception hall where a long, lace-covered banquet table displayed the beautiful multitiered wedding cake, the crystal punch bowl and cups, sterling silverware, and frou-frou monogrammed napkins. The only problem was that whoever set up the table had forgotten to fasten the latch on one of the folding legs. As soon as the red punch was poured into the crystal punch bowl, the leg buckled and everything slid down to the end of the table and onto the floor with a clatter! The cake toppled amid the pool of red punch and the napkins were soaked. Everyone looked to the bride and groom, expecting shock and horror. To everyone's delight, however, Kevin and Ruth broke out into hysterical laughter!

But it's no laughing matter when one of the "legs" of our sexuality buckles, because then our lives can become a slippery slope leading to discontentment, sexual compromise, self-loathing, and emotional brokenness. When this happens, the blessing that God intended to bring richness and pleasure to our lives feels more like a curse that brings great pain and despair.

As I mentioned, our sexuality is comprised of four distinct aspects: the physical, mental, emotional, and spiritual dimensions of our being. These four parts combine to form the unique individual that God designed you to be. Most people make the mistake of assuming that our sexuality is limited to the physical, that we are "sexual" only when we are having sex. Nothing could be further from the truth. God designed all humans as sexual beings, whether they ever have sex or not. You were sexual the day you were conceived. You were sexual when you dressed your Barbie dolls and when you cried over your first broken heart. You are even being sexual right now as you are reading this book.

By definition, our sexuality isn't *what we do.* Even people who are committed to celibacy are sexual beings. Our sexuality is *who we are,* and we were made with a body, mind, heart, and spirit, not just a body. Therefore, sexual integrity is not just about physical chastity. It is about purity in all four aspects of our being (body, mind, heart, and spirit). When all four aspects line up perfectly, our "tabletop" (our life) reflects balance and integrity.

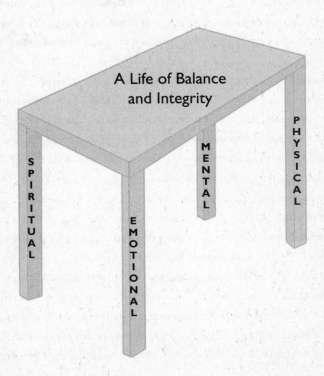

UNIDENTIFIED SLIPPERY SLOPES

Have there ever been seasons of your life when you focused a great deal on one of these aspects (physical, mental, emotional, or spiritual), but completely neglected another one? Let me show you what I mean:

- Nicole, a lawyer, has been doing research for months on a big case she is litigating but has made little time for socializing, exercising, or spending quality time with her husband. (Nicole is overfeeding the mental aspect while starving the emotional and physical.)

- Michelle spends a great deal of time volunteering at the church, teaching women's Bible studies, and serving on the intercessory prayer team, but she has little interest in having sex with her husband. (Michelle is overfeeding the spiritual while neglecting the physical.)

- Ann masturbates often, and sex usually becomes a part of her dating relationships. As a result, her guilt keeps her from attending church regularly or reading her Bible. (Ann is overfeeding the physical while starving the spiritual.)

- Theresa frequently compares her husband to other men, which not only leads her to fantasize about these other men's showing an interest in her, but also causes her to resist her husband's advances due to the disillusionment and disappointment she feels. (Theresa is overfeeding the mental and emotional with a false, fantasized sense of intimacy—which is actually the equivalent to neglecting it—as well as neglecting the physical.)

These women are unsatisfied and are sexually and emotionally unfulfilled. They live unbalanced lives and lack sexual integrity, even though some are avoiding sex altogether. You see, just as sexuality isn't defined by *what we do* but by *who we are*, sexual integrity isn't defined as "not sleeping around" or "keeping our panties on," but as having a perfect balance between the physical, mental, emotional, and spiritual dimensions of our being.

In order to have ultimate fulfillment and feel that physical, mental, emotional, and spiritual stability that God intended for us to have, we have to attend to each leg of our table according to God's perfect plan. If one leg is neglected, abused, or attended to in an unrighteous manner, the result is some sort of sexual compromise or emotional brokenness. When each leg is attended to or fulfilled righteously, the result is sexual integrity and emotional wholeness. If you are wondering how to accomplish this state of balance and wholeness, rest assured that, by the time you get to the end of this book, you will have the answers.

For a single woman, sexual integrity equates to trying at all costs to avoid feeding any physical, mental, emotional, or spiritual longings for a man that cannot be fulfilled righteously. She looks to God to satisfy these needs until she has a husband to make these connections with. It doesn't mean she can't be interested in or hopeful of having a husband, but that she tries with all her might to save her body, mind, heart, and spirit for the man she marries.

For a married woman, sexual integrity equates to intimately connecting physically, mentally, emotionally, and spiritually (in all ways, not just some) with her husband and no other man outside of her marriage. Any compromise whatsoever (physical, mental, emotional, or spiritual) affects her sexual integrity as a whole. One infected part will eventually infect all of its corresponding parts or, at the very least, rob her of the sexual wholeness and fulfillment that God longs for her to have.

The problem with most of our plans to remain sexually pure or faithful within marriage is that they only include physical boundaries. Rarely do we understand the emotional progression of relationships before it's too late and we've been sucked into an affair of the heart. Because a woman can jeopardize her emotional integrity long before her body becomes vulnerable to temptation, I encourage women to focus on keeping their emotions in check (the topic of chapter 6). When we guard our hearts and keep them pure and faithful, we will protect our bodies as well.

But most of us didn't know this as we were growing up. As young women, we pushed the envelope while we were dating. Kissing on the first date was almost an expectation. Allowing him to go to first, second, or even third "base" was considered okay, as long as he couldn't proclaim to his friends that he'd hit a "home run" with you. But all of this sexual activity during dating didn't prepare us for true love, lifetime commitments, and faithful marriages as we thought it would. Instead, it prepared us to crave the intensity and excitement that only a new relationship brings, causing us to be discontent once we marry and the relationship ages.

When we enter marriage as "technical virgins" (having experienced most sexual pleasures with the exception of intercourse), we often face overwhelming temptations to act out sexually with another man without understanding why. The reason is simply because we never learned to nip these temptations in the bud when we were single. Because we never learned sexual self-control as single women (not just physical, but emotional, mental, and spiritual self-control), it seems extremely difficult to exercise it with the added stressors of two kids, a minivan, and a mortgage payment. How disappointing to discover that the wedding band placed on our finger didn't change us at all!

A COVENANT WITH THE EYES OF YOUR HEART

If reading about tabletop sexuality and the need for perfect balance between the physical, mental, emotional, and spiritual dimensions of our being made you feel uneasy or convicted you, I encourage you to make a covenant similar to the one discussed in *Every Man's Battle*. Many men, after reading *Every Man's Battle,* are making a covenant with their eyes similar to the one Job made when he said, "I made a covenant with my eyes not to look lustfully at a girl" (Job 31:1). While most women don't lust after men's bodies (although there are certainly exceptions to this rule), we cross the line of sexual integrity in other ways. When we engage in emotional affairs, mental fantasies, and unhealthy comparisons, we are crossing the line of sexual integrity and undermining God's plan to grant us ultimate sexual and emotional fulfillment with our (current or future) husbands. We need to make a covenant with the eyes of our hearts not to look at other people (real or imagined) to fulfill our emotional needs and desires in ways that compromise our sexual integrity, whether we are married or single.

What kind of boundaries do you have in place to protect your heart, mind, and spirit in addition to your body? If you've never really thought them through, chapters 5 through 8 will help you do just that, but for now let's look at the standard of integrity to which God calls us.

LEGALISM VS. LOVE

In discussing sexual integrity, most women want a list of dos and don'ts, cans and can'ts, shoulds and shouldn'ts. They want to know: "What can I get away with? How far can I go? What's too far?"

The problem with these questions is that they are based on what is culturally and socially acceptable, which changes from place to place and from decade to decade. In our culture we see nothing wrong with having close friends of the opposite sex. However, in biblical times a woman couldn't remove the veil from her face for anyone other than her husband. In the Western world, women often go out of their way to get a man's attention. In the Middle Eastern countries, women walk several paces behind the men and try to go unnoticed. Today American and European women want to know how short their skirts, shorts, or tops can be, but it wasn't that long ago that the issue of open-toed shoes was creating quite the scandal among Christians. Could you imagine a *sandal scandal* in your church today?

Therefore, a list of laws about what women of integrity can and can't wear, should and shouldn't do and say, and so on, isn't the answer. What we need is a standard of sexual integrity that will withstand the test of time as well as apply to all women of all cultures. But how can we develop a set of rules that are timeless and all-inclusive?

The answer lies not in legalism but in Christian love. Of the plethora of rules and regulations set out in the Old Testament, God boiled them all down to just ten commandments. Then in the New Testament, Jesus reduced all those laws down to only two. If we can simply learn to live by these two commandments, we can live a life of sexual integrity.

These two laws are explained when Jesus responded to the question, "Which is the greatest commandment?"

"Love the Lord your God with all your heart and with all your soul and with all your mind." This is the first and greatest commandment. And the second is like it: "Love your neighbor as yourself." All the Law and the Prophets hang on these two commandments. (Matthew 22:37-40)

Jesus was saying that the law isn't what is important. Love is what is important. If we love God, love our neighbor, and love ourselves (in that order), then we can live far above any set of rules or regulations. We have freedom to live apart from any legalistic standards when we live by the spirit of love. Paul echoed this form of "freedom with responsibility" when he wrote:

> "Everything is permissible"—but not everything is beneficial. "Everything is permissible"—but not everything is constructive. Nobody should seek his own good, but the good of others. (1 Corinthians 10:23-24)

Paul was saying that you can do most anything, but it isn't always in your best interest or in the interest of others. Focus not on what is "allowed," but on what is best for all involved. How can we apply this freedom to sexual integrity? Pick any issue and sift it through this "law vs. love" filter:

- While it is lawful for a married woman to flirt with a man, is it a truly loving thing to do? While it is lawful for a single woman to flirt with a married man, is it the loving thing to do? (Will it benefit him in a righteous way?)
- There is no law against flattering clothes, but is our motive in wearing them to build others up or to build up our ego?

QUESTIONS OF COMPROMISE *Don't Ask*	QUESTIONS OF INTEGRITY *Do Ask*
• Are my actions lawful?	• Are my actions loving to others?
• Will anyone find out?	• Is this something I'd be proud of?
• Would anyone condemn me?	• Is this my highest standard?
• Is this socially acceptable?	• Is this in line with my convictions?
• Are my clothes too revealing?	• Am I dressing for attention?
• How can I get what I want?	• What is my motive for wanting this?
• Can I get away with saying this?	• Would this be better left unsaid?
• Will this hurt anyone?	• Will this benefit others?

Figure 2.2

- We have freedom of speech in this country, but are the words we choose in the best interest of the men we speak to or do they support our own private agenda?
- Do our thoughts seek the highest good for others, or do they serve our own dysfunctional needs and emotional cravings?
- Is the attention and affection we may want to express to a man going to edify him or cause him to stumble and fall into temptation?

We must look beyond the movements to the motivations behind our actions. By doing this, we no longer have to concern ourselves with the law because we are acting by a higher standard, a standard of love. Figure 2.2 shows the difference between evaluating our motives and behaviors through the lens of legalism and evaluating them through the lens of love.

We are each held accountable by God for what we know to do. If we want to gain the prize of sexual integrity, we may need to let go of some of our "freedoms" (in dress, thoughts, speech, and behavior) in order to serve the best interest of others out of love. Not only will God provide this knowledge of how to act with integrity, He will also honor those who apply this knowledge and act with responsibility.

A WOMAN OF SEXUAL INTEGRITY

Let's put this all together. For a Christian woman, sexual and emotional integrity means that her thoughts, words, emotions, and actions all reflect an inner beauty and a sincere love for God, others, and herself. This doesn't mean she is never tempted to think, say, feel, or do something inappropriate, but that she tries diligently to resist these temptations and stands firm in her convictions. She doesn't use men in an attempt to get her emotional cravings met or entertain sexual or romantic fantasies about men she is not married to. She doesn't compare her husband to other men, discounting his personal worth and withholding a part of herself from him as punishment for his imperfections. She doesn't dress to seek male attention, but she doesn't limit herself to a wardrobe of ankle-length muumuus, either. She may dress fashionably and look sharp or may even appear sexy (like beauty, sexy is in the eye of the beholder), but her motivation isn't self-seeking or seductive. She presents herself as an attractive woman because she knows she represents God to others.

A woman of integrity lives a life that lines up with her Christian beliefs. She lives according to the standard of love rather than law. She does not claim to be a follower of Christ yet disregard His many teachings on sexual immorality, lustful thoughts, immodest dress, and inappropriate talk. A woman of integrity lives what she believes about God, and it shows everywhere from the boardroom to the bedroom.

If you are ready to discover more about how you can claim the prize of sexual integrity, keep reading as we dispel some of the most popular myths that keep women entrenched in this battle.

 Therefore I do not run like a [woman] running aimlessly; I do not fight like a [woman] beating the air. No, I beat my body [and my mind] and make it my slave so that after I have preached to others, I myself will not be disqualified for the prize.

—*1 Corinthians 9:26-27*

seven myths that intensify our struggle

Wisdom is better than weapons of war.

ECCLESIASTES 9:18

In my thirteen years of speaking and lay counseling with women on sexual issues, I've uncovered seven popular myths that I believe confuse the issue and make sexual integrity far more challenging. Although at first glance you may not believe that you subscribe to a particular misconception, I encourage you to read about it anyway. We are often only aware of what we believe in regard to the things we have actually experienced but are undecided about our beliefs regarding the things or feelings we have not yet experienced. If we understand these myths and the lies they are based on, we'll have a stronger defense if and when we're tempted in one of these areas.

MYTH 1

There's nothing wrong with comparing myself or my husband to other people.

While it is common knowledge that women often compare themselves to one another and compare their husbands to other men, you may ask, "What has that got to do with sexual and emotional integrity?" To answer this question, let's first go back to our definition of a woman of integrity: Her thoughts, words, emotions, and actions all reflect an inner beauty and sincere love for God, others, and herself.

When we compare ourselves to others, we put one person above the other. We either come out on top (producing vanity and pride in our lives), or we come up short (producing feelings of disappointment with what God gave us). Regardless of how we measure up when we make these comparisons, our motives are selfish and sinful rather than loving.

Let's be honest. When we compare ourselves to the large woman we saw in the cookie aisle, we may waltz through the parking lot with our groceries, feeling good about ourselves because we feel thin. We feel attractive. We may even feel powerful. If our obsession with our body continues, we may even open the door to further temptations. We may experience a yearning to prove that we are more attractive than other women. Some have taken this to the extreme by landing in bed with their best friend's husband. How does this happen? It begins in a mind obsessed with comparison.

Or perhaps the opposite scenario plays itself out: We walk through the produce section and notice the local ballet teacher squeezing the organic tomatoes. We look at her perky breasts and tight behind, and we feel like an overripe watermelon. We feel huge and sloppy. We feel powerless. We wonder who would ever want to be with us. Such feelings can lead us to become victims of seduction. When we focus so much on superficial appearances, our self-esteem can become so low that if a man takes notice of us, we are pleasantly surprised and become affirmation-seeking missiles. We begin to hunger for a man's approval so much that his flattery and attention can manipulate us.

Not only can we attract unhealthy relationships with men when we feel intimidated by or superior to other women, we also miss out on something we all desperately need: intimacy with our sisters. Whether we are single or married, our sisters often keep us connected to God's love in a way that a boyfriend or husband can't or won't. If we could stop competing and start connecting with other women, this battle for sexual and emotional integrity wouldn't be nearly as overwhelming. Remaining connected to healthy, loving friendships can keep us out of bed with the next guy we meet and help us satisfy our longing for emotional fulfillment.

In addition to comparing ourselves with other women, some of us compare our husbands to other men. Here are a few examples of statements I've heard from women who have obviously fallen into this trap:

- "I wish my husband aged as well as Sean Connery!"
- "My husband is far from being a rocket scientist or brain surgeon, you know!"
- "My husband just doesn't meet my emotional needs like my coworker does."
- "You are so lucky to have a husband who will go to church with you every Sunday."

When women compare their husbands with other men, they are toying with a threat similar to the threat a man plays with when visually lusting after other women. Whether the comparison is physical, mental, emotional, or spiritual, we not only show disrespect for our husband's uniqueness, but also undermine our marriage and our emotional integrity. Comparisons can lead women to wonder, *Why does my husband have to be like this? Why can't he be more like so-and-so?*

Sometimes a woman will fall further into this trap by entertaining more and more thoughts of so-and-so until her fantasy life becomes a world that she escapes to in order to make herself feel more valuable and loved. In her fantasy life, she deserves someone more handsome, more intelligent, more emotionally attentive or more spiritual than she has in reality. At the very least, when a woman's comparisons of her husband with other men heightens any disappointment or disillusionment she feels with her own husband, it can prevent her from getting excited about him sexually or emotionally. These comparisons encourage her once-glowing passion for her husband to fade to a mere tolerance of him as she forgets all about the wonderful man she fell in love with.

Let's face it, there will always be men more handsome, intelligent, sensitive, or spiritual than our husbands, just as there will always be women slimmer, smarter, wittier, or holier than we are. If "others" are the measuring stick that we use to place value on ourselves or on those we love, then we are doing exactly what Paul warns against in 2 Corinthians 10:12: "When they measure themselves by themselves and compare themselves with themselves, they are not wise." However, God gives us grace to accept our husbands and ourselves as we really are, and He gives us the ability to truly love one another unconditionally and unreservedly.

If we crave genuine intimacy, we must learn to seek it only in this kind of grace-filled relationship. The word *intimacy* itself can be best defined by breaking it into syllables, *in-to-me-see*. Can we see into each other and respect, appreciate, and value what is really there, regardless of how that measures up to anyone else? That is what unconditional love and relational intimacy is all about, and this type of intimacy can be discovered only by two people who are seeking sexual and emotional integrity with all their mind, body, heart, and soul.

MYTH 2

I am mature enough to watch any movie or television show, read any book, listen to any music, or surf any Web sites without being affected in a negative way.

Most of us become desensitized to what we see or hear. I've demonstrated this through an experiment I conduct when teaching about sexuality during weekend retreats for youth groups. I once recorded two hours of prime-time television shows such as *Friends* and *Seinfeld,* then edited the tape down to a twelve-minute clip including only the sexual innuendos (anything visual or auditory related to inappropriate sexual conduct). As I show this video clip, I challenge the audience to keep count during these twelve minutes of how many sexual messages they see or hear, giving me a sign (placing their thumb on their nose) to indicate that they recognize each one.

As many times as I have conducted this experiment, I'm amazed at how the same thing happens every time. They catch maybe the first three or four innuendos, but then become so engrossed in the funny scenes that they forget to give me the sign or to keep count. At the end of the twelve minutes, I ask, "How many did you count?" The average response? Eleven or twelve. The actual number of visual or verbal innuendos? Forty-one.

Even the adults in the room do not usually recognize more than 50 percent of these innuendos because they are so accustomed to crass humor. As a society, we have become so desensitized by sexual messages that we often unscrew our heads, put them under the Lazy-Boy recliner, and tolerantly allow the television to fill our minds with worldly scripts. Once our minds are corrupted, our hearts memorize these scripts, and then they seep into our lives.

Jesus taught his disciples this principle in the gospel of Luke when He said: "The good [woman] brings good things out of the good stored up in [her] heart, and the evil [woman] brings evil things out of the evil stored up in [her] heart" (6:45).

Everything you choose to take in through your mind can be stored up in your heart, and it is your heart that determines the direction you will take and the choices you will make in the future when confronted with temptation. If you fill your mind with images of sexually compromising comments and situations, you will become desensitized to similar scenarios in your own life.

A good rule of thumb is never to watch a movie or television program or read a book that you wouldn't want others to know about. If you have to keep it a secret, chances are it's going to greatly intensify your battle for sexual integrity and undermine your ultimate fulfillment.

You should also be careful about how you use the Internet. I am very thankful that I reached a place of sexual and emotional integrity before the days of e-mails and chat rooms. So many women tell me how they were sucked into a living nightmare through the World Wide Web, falling head over heels for men they initially thought were their Prince Charmings, only to discover they were frogs with lots and lots of warts.

What makes chat rooms so alluring to women? Here are some of the answers I've received, along with my rebuttal:

- *It is exciting to be intimate with a stranger.* Since when is sitting at a desk and typing back and forth *intimate?* And anyone can be excited by a stranger. Everything you learn or share is new, but learning new things about a strange person is not intimacy. Intimacy is seeing what is *truly* on the inside of a person (which can only be discovered face to face over long periods of time such as what you experience in marriage). Be careful not to mistake *intensity* for *intimacy.* Intensity fades as the newness wears off, but intimacy continues to blossom the longer you know a person.

- *I can be anyone I want to be while online.* Why would you want to waste your time being anyone other than yourself? You could spend that time becoming the person that God wants you to be. Besides, if you aren't yourself, how can you feel good about this man's feelings for you? You can't even be sure he knows you. Also remember that he can be anybody he wants to be too. He can act like Regis Philbin but turn out to be more like Jack the Ripper!

- *I appreciate someone being interested in getting to know me regardless of what I look like.* But don't think for a minute that he's not eventually going to be very interested in what you look like. Then what will you do? Why go there? Don't get hooked.

- *I enjoy just conversing with a man without having the expectation placed on me to get physical.* You may not want to get physical with him now, but after you've swallowed every line he's fed you about himself and poured your heart out to him, you are going to want to move beyond the emotional. Remember, women are Crock-Pots who love to simmer emotionally, but once we've had time to warm up, we get *hot!* To avoid getting burned, I suggest befriending only real people in our lives (not virtual people).

MYTH 3

It doesn't hurt anyone if I fantasize about someone other than my husband when we make love.

Just as wives have the right to be offended by their husbands' wandering eyes, men have the right to be offended by their wives' wandering minds. For women, orgasm is probably 10 percent physical and 90 percent mental. If your husband is trying to please you, he can forget about it if your mind is a million miles away, say on your grocery list. A woman must focus mentally on the sexual experience in order to derive ultimate pleasure from it.

Unfortunately, some women focus on the wrong things during these passionate moments. They entertain thoughts of someone else. They place themselves in the middle of the plot of the romance novel they are reading. They usher in flashbacks from old lovers, previous graphic scenes they were exposed to through romance novels or pornography, or images of the latest Hollywood heartthrob. Such images rob us of the intimacy that we crave. When you fantasize about someone else when making love with your husband, you are mentally making love with another man. *He,* not your husband, is the one you feel passionate about. *He,* not your husband, is the one you feel close to emotionally.

Sex between a husband and wife was meant to be the most intimate thing this side of heaven and can be even more fulfilling than any fantasy imaginable. Ironically, many of the women who tell me that they regularly think of another man while making love to their husbands also tell me that they feel guilty, empty, dissatisfied, and confused.

While it is normal and healthy to have fantasies, they need to be restricted to your marriage partner. It's okay to fantasize that he brings you flowers or makes you a candlelight dinner or rubs lotion on your back. It's okay to fantasize about showering together or having wild sex on some tropical deserted island—as long as it is with your husband! Sharing these appropriate fantasies with your spouse will add passion and sizzle to your relationship. However, fantasizing about anyone else is mental and emotional unfaithfulness to your husband. Even if you convince yourself that you would never act on the fantasies that include someone outside of your marriage, remember that God looks at the heart (1 Samuel 16:7), and His heart breaks when yours is divided, even if only in your fantasies.

MYTH 4

Thinking about what kind of man I'd like to have if my husband were to die is not a big deal, as long as I am not plotting how to carry that out!

"I wonder if he'll die first so I can have some chance at a happier future." I'm amazed at how many women have confessed pondering this secret thought. While some women are horrified that they would ever think such a thing, others can laugh at the thought. Samantha is one of the latter, confessing that she has almost the same mental conversation with herself each time her husband is late coming home from the office.

She explains:

I'm usually standing in the kitchen preparing dinner right at 6 P.M. I'm constantly watching the clock, expecting Frank to walk in any minute. He's so punctual I can almost set my clock to his walking in the door, sniffing to see what's cooking. He's also very considerate to call when he is running late. But I confess that there have been several times that 6:05 came around and I was concerned. By 6:10, I'm worried. By 6:15, I'm frantic. As I continue cooking, ideas roll through my mind: *There's probably been a car accident. I wonder if he's dead? A policeman will probably show up in a little while to bring me his personal effects. How will I break it to the kids? Can I be strong for them? What kind of flowers will I put on the casket? Yellow lilies were always his favorite. Oh, and I'll have the soloist sing his favorite hymn, "How Great Thou Art." Will I be able to keep the checkbook balanced on my own? Will I remember to keep the oil changed in the car? I wonder how much life insurance he's left me? I wonder how long it will be before I begin dating again? And when I do, who would I want to go out with? Dan. Oh, I'm just crazy about Dan. I don't know why anyone hasn't snatched him up before now. He's so witty and charming. And such a godly man! He'd make a great stepfather to the kids. I'm sure they will love him as much as I do. It will be hard getting over Frank, but I think it will all be okay...*

Suddenly the door opens and in walks Frank with a sheepish look on his face. "Sorry I'm late, honey! I had to stop at the hardware store and I didn't have my cell phone with me."

I tell him (with a hidden twinge of disappointment), "Oh, it's okay, dear. I was just finishing up dinner."

You may be laughing at Samantha's antics, but ask yourself, "Does this sound familiar?" Do you go through these mental gymnastics and find yourself wondering, *Will my next husband be any more attentive? More fun? More financially stable? More spiritual? More interested in my sexual pleasure?* Do you get excited when you allow your mind to wander in this direction?

While it is normal to think about what you would do if your husband were to die before you, mentally moving on to the next husband and entertaining thoughts of a more fulfilling future as a result of his death crosses the line of sexual and emotional integrity. I recommend that you discern why you are thinking in this direction. Do any of these motives sound painfully familiar? If so, you may be compromising your sexual integrity to the point that you are seriously damaging yourself and your marriage relationship.

- Pride—*I deserve better.*
- Rejection—*Maybe the next one will appreciate me more than this one.*
- Lust—*I hope the next one will be more sexy.*
- Selfishness—*I'll be able to enjoy my life a little more without having to cater to him.*
- Laziness—*I'm tired of trying to communicate with him. He's a brick wall. I'll just have to accept that he will never meet my needs and hope that the next husband is more understanding.*

If, because you aren't happy in your marriage, you daydream about who you might marry should your husband die, be warned. You are likely to encounter the same disappointments and problems if you remarry. Regardless of how great "the next guy" may be should you ever find yourself widowed (or divorced), remember that there is a common denominator in these multiple marriages—you. If you cannot conquer pride, feelings of rejection, lust, selfishness, and laziness in this relationship and communicate your needs in such a way that inspires your husband to fill your emotional bank account, you can be sure that a different man isn't the remedy.

Put all your eggs in one basket. Invest in the relationship you've got. Focus on your marriage wholeheartedly, as if no other man existed. Assume that your spouse is the man you will grow old with. Your husband is God's gift to you. Unwrap the gift and enjoy him for as long as you have him.

MYTH 5

Masturbation does not hurt me, my relationship with my (current or future) husband, or my relationship with God.

If a married woman masturbates without her husband's knowledge, or if a married or single woman masturbates entertaining thoughts of someone who is not her husband, I believe that her behavior undermines her integrity and even her ulti-mate sexual and emotional fulfillment.

Many single women tell me I cannot expect them *not* to masturbate. They say things like, "I must have a physical sexual release, and if I can't have sex then I have to masturbate." Believe it or not, no one ever died from not having an orgasm. From the reports I've received from women, the momentary stress relief masturbating may provide may not be worth the long-term stress that the habit creates.

Denise told me:

> I sometimes masturbate before going out on dates so that I won't cave in
> to sexual temptations. But then I think during the evening about how
> unsatisfied I still feel and how lonely it is not to have someone else in-
> volved. I often give in and have sex out of disappointment with the mas-
> turbation experience. Then I feel guilty about both. I just wish I had more
> self-control.

Masturbation hurts Denise. It serves only to fuel her sexual fire, not quench it. It's likely that she even imagined herself being sexually involved with the man she was going out with. When we think about doing something and play it out in our thoughts, it makes it that much easier to engage in the behavior. If a woman can-not control herself while alone, what hope does she have when some smooth-talking hunk of a man starts whispering sweet nothings in her ear?

Also, no lust can ever be satisfied; once you begin feeding baby monsters, their appetites grow bigger and they require *more!* You are better off never feeding those monsters in the first place. As my friend says, "If sin doesn't know you, it won't call your name!" Once the sin of masturbation does know you by name, it *will* call. And call…and call…and call.

Heather e-mails:

> When I was in sixth grade, I had a friend spend the night and we bathed
> together. She showed me how to masturbate, and I've been habitually mas-
> turbating ever since. I feel like I cannot control myself, and it brings so much

guilt. I struggle with sexual thoughts, allowing myself to become aroused just by thinking about masturbating. I have taken this before the Lord so many times. What can I do? This has been something that makes me feel so dirty and inferior, but even knowing this doesn't seem to be enough to make me stop.

The only way to kill a bad habit is to *starve it to death*. Starving a bad habit can be painful, but not as painful as letting it rule over you. This is why Peter warned, "Dear friends, I urge you, as aliens and strangers in the world, to abstain from sinful desires, which war against your soul" (1 Peter 2:11).

Many married women continue in their addiction to masturbation even after they have the freedom of sexual expression with their mate. They can't see what this habit does to their marriage. But think about it. You train your body as well as your mind as to what it finds pleasurable and how to orgasm, and masturbation trains a woman to "fly solo." This can cause problems because your husband may not know how to please you in the same way, which could make your marital sex life very frustrating and disappointing to the both of you. Most husbands find pleasure and satisfaction in bringing their wives to orgasm. If you typically find sexual release through masturbation, you may rob your husband of this pleasure by insisting that he allow you to "help him." If you cannot imagine how this will make your husband feel, imagine how you'd feel if you were making love, and within a short time your husband said, "Thanks, honey, but you are going to have to let me take it from here." Feel rejected? Wonder what is wrong with you and what you are not doing right? He will feel exactly the same way if you have to masturbate in order to reach an orgasm.

Even if your husband's touch can bring you to orgasm without masturbation, if you are in the habit of fantasizing about someone or something else in order to "get there" (similar to what is mentally required when you masturbate), you rob yourself of genuine sexual intimacy with your husband. Quinn admits:

I was disappointed in our sex life when I got married. I expected that my husband would have the same magic touch that I had with myself, but he is rougher and more aggressive than I am used to. I've tried to teach him what I like, but one night after I tried to coach him he politely told me, "Why don't you just do it yourself if you don't like the way I do it?" On the one hand I was relieved that I could finally do what felt good to me, but on the other hand I know it must be a blow to his ego that I'm not as aroused by his touch as I am by my own.

Often women who want to stop masturbating (be it for reasons of integrity in singleness or for relational intimacy in marriage) discover that, rather than controlling their desires, their desires control them. They find themselves compulsively masturbating, unable to stop even though they are aware that it is an unhealthy habit. Stephen Arterburn explains in his book *Addicted to Love* how self-gratification becomes self-destructive:

> Compulsive masturbation, built on fantasy [and/or] pornography, is an escape from intimacy. A person who is a compulsive masturbator will be unable to experience genuine intimacy. Sex becomes a one-sided process of self-gratification. The addict would rather masturbate than take the time to develop a relationship. Expecting marriage to eliminate the drive to masturbate, the addict soon finds that intimate sex is too much trouble and returns to the compulsion.
>
> Everyone needs to be nurtured, to feel loved, to feel love toward another. But love is risky. Love holds the possibility of rejection or disappointment. The masturbator finds it easier to fall back on self-gratification. What seems to many like a harmless habit becomes a trap that blocks out others and forces the addict to suffer alone.[1]

The most popular argument in favor of self-gratification is, "The Bible does not expressly forbid it." Let's be honest. When women masturbate, they don't think pure thoughts, and the Bible is very clear about that issue (see Philippians 4:8). We don't entertain thoughts that are pure, noble, or praiseworthy when we engage in self-gratification. Women who masturbate have some fantasy about another person, some scenario, some ritual they play out in their minds in order to reach an orgasm. But what does Paul have to say about such things?

Put to death, therefore, whatever belongs to your earthly nature: sexual immorality, impurity, lust, evil desires and greed, which is idolatry. Because of these, the wrath of God is coming. (Colossians 3:5-6)

It is God's will that you should be sanctified: that you should avoid sexual immorality; that each of you should learn to control [her] own body in a way that is holy and honorable, not in passionate lust like the heathen, who do not know God. (1 Thessalonians 4:3-5)

Scripture also says that some things that may be permissible are still not beneficial (1 Corinthians 10:23). Masturbation enslaves you and brings you into bondage. I believe that is enough reason to abstain from the practice all together.

Finally, masturbation is a very proud response to our human desires. Such actions tell God, "You can't satisfy me nor is your Holy Spirit strong enough to control me. I must take care of my own physical desires." Do you hear the pride in that attitude? Do you sense the rejection of God's sovereignty and ability to help you in your time of need?

God made every fiber and every nerve of our bodies, and He can satisfy every fiber and nerve as well. He knows how you feel and what you need better than you know yourself. He knows what will truly satisfy you—and it's not orgasm, particularly orgasm achieved through masturbation and impure thoughts. It may feel good for the moment, but it doesn't bring lasting satisfaction. That can only be found in relationship. God wants a close, intimate relationship with you. Once you allow Him to prove Himself in this area, you will understand that self-gratification was really never any gratification at all. Striving for God-gratification instead of self-gratification will ensure that your body, mind, heart, and spirit remain pure.

Who may ascend the hill of the LORD?
    Who may stand in his holy place?
[She] who has clean hands and a pure heart,
    who does not lift up [her] soul to an idol
    or swear by what is false. (Psalm 24:3-4)

MYTH 6

Because I feel so sexually tempted, I must already be guilty, so why bother resisting?

Satan's favorite strategy for convincing women to cross the line between temptation and sin is false guilt. If sexual integrity is a battle you are entrenched in, you've probably had some of these thoughts rolling around in your head until you can no longer think straight:

- *You can't deny that you want him! You may as well go after him!*
- *You know you'll never be able to be faithful to one man forever!*
- *You've already gone this far, what's one step further?*
- *You've thought about this moment for months! Don't back out now!*
- *If you want to keep him, you are going to have to give him what he wants!*

These lies are temptations from the enemy, not evidence that you are already guilty! I call this false guilt because temptation, in and of itself, is *not* sin. There's nothing to feel guilty about when you are tempted. If you don't believe me, maybe you will believe the writer of Hebrews when he says:

> For we do not have a high priest who is unable to sympathize with our weaknesses, but we have one who has been tempted in every way, just as we are—yet was without sin. Let us then approach the throne of grace with confidence, so that we may receive mercy and find grace to help us in our time of need. (Hebrews 4:15-16)

Did you get that? Jesus himself was tempted in every way! "Even sexually?" you say. Why not sexually? He was a man in every sense of the word. He had beautiful women following Him around and taking care of His needs with their own money. He was reaching out to minister to women who would have loved to have Jesus hold them in His arms. The writer didn't say, "He was tempted in every way except sexually." He was human in every way and experienced every human temptation. He set the example for us that just because we are tempted does not mean that we must give in and become a slave to our passions.

But women often make the mistake of believing that because they are so attracted to someone, they will inevitably fall into a relationship with that person, regardless of how inappropriate that relationship may be. As you will see in chapter 6, women can draw a line between attraction and acting out on that attraction. It is normal to feel attracted to multiple people. It is not normal to *attach* yourself to multiple people. Remember that love is not a feeling, but a commitment. You've not broken your commitment to your husband if you feel tempted to seek satisfaction outside your marriage, but only when you've allowed yourself to stray there and stay there mentally, emotionally, or physically.

MYTH 7

There's no one who would really understand my struggle.

I believe that this myth exists because women don't usually discuss their sex lives with other women, perhaps because they fear judgment. Unfortunately, these fears are often confirmed as legitimate very early in childhood when you trust a grade-school friend with a secret and she inevitably whispers it to two friends, or worse, tells the boy you have a crush on all about your confession. These experiences taught us that we must guard our deepest, darkest secrets from other women.

Some of us grew up with guys as our best friends because we felt so strongly that girls simply could not be trusted. Many of us also found out the hard way that confiding in a young man could even be more dangerous than confiding in a female friend. All a girl could do is betray your confidence. A boy could take advantage of your vulnerability and make you his next prey if you weren't standing firm in your convictions.

Another reason women aren't as open about their sexual struggles is because of the humiliation that comes with giving sex in order to get love. Most women don't brag about the number of sexual partners they've had. That's because for a woman the relationship is the prize; the sex was simply the price she had to pay to get the prize. If she paid the price, but still didn't get the prize, there is an incredible amount of humiliation that comes with that. What woman wants to announce to the world her humiliation?

Maybe if we knew how common these struggles are to women, it would remove some of the stigma behind having these kinds of "issues." According to Dr. Tim Clinton, president of the American Association of Christian Counselors, 67 percent of all women will experience at least one or more premarital or extra-marital affair in her lifetime.[2] That is the number of women who *give in* to these temptations. I believe the percentage is much higher (I'm guessing in the 90 per-cent range) of those women who simply experience the temptation to engage in premarital or extramarital affairs.

Paul tells us in 1 Corinthians 10:13, "No temptation has seized you except what is common to [woman]. And God is faithful; he will not let you be tempted beyond what you can bear. But when you are tempted, he will also provide a way out so that you can stand up under it." Paul didn't say, "If you experience sexual temptation, there must be something wrong with you because no one else struggles with it that much." He said that all temptations are common. And because God creates all human beings (regardless of gender, nationality, or economic back-ground) as sexual human beings, you can bet that sexual and relational tempta-tions are by far the most common temptations on the planet.

What "way out" does God usually provide so that we can stand up under the temptation? Does He turn off our emotions altogether? No. Does He make the object of our desire fall off the face of the earth? No. My experience has been that the way out is usually provided through an accountability friendship with another woman who can sympathize with my weakness and encourage me to stand firm in the face of battle. As I give a trusted confidant permission to ask me the hard, per-sonal questions and speak the truth in love (even if it hurts), I am required to examine the condition of my heart and mind much more than if I harbor these things within myself. And when I fail to live up to God's standards, an account-ability friend will sharpen me, not with harsh judgment but with a reminder to use good judgment. As I have confessed certain temptations to trusted friends and asked for accountability, I've learned that I am truly not alone in my struggles.

In *Every Man's Battle*, Stephen Arterburn and Fred Stoeker describe the per-centages of men who struggle with sexual issues using the following "bell curve" analogy:

Another way of looking at the scope of the problem is to picture a bell curve. According to our experiences, we figure around 10 percent of men have no sexual-temptation problem with their eyes and their minds. At the other end of the curve, we figure there's another 10 percent of men who are sexual addicts and have a serious problem with lust. They've been so beaten and scarred by emotional events that they simply can't overcome that sin in their lives. They need more counseling and a transforming washing by the Word. The rest of us comprise the middle 80 percent, living in various shades of gray when it comes to sexual sin.[3]

I believe the same illustration is true for women. There may be 10 percent of us who are the June Cleaver type of gal who is as pure as the driven snow and would never dream of longing after any other man besides Ward. Then there are perhaps another 10 percent of us who are the Playboy Bunny type of girl, constantly tossing out innuendos, shooting seductive glances, and enjoying the spoils of war. The rest of us probably fall into that 80 percent range that struggle with sexual and emotional integrity by varying degrees.

Thinking you are the only one who feels overwhelmed by sexual temptations will make you more vulnerable for failure because you will be less likely to ask for help to change. If this is your struggle, you can benefit from genuine intimacy in female friendships. This is something I've come to depend on in my quest to maintain sexual integrity. Your friends can offer you a lifeline to hold on to when the temptation gets too deep to stand alone.

WINNING THE BATTLE WITH TRUTH

If any of these myths awakened you to the fact that you are standing in the line of fire in this struggle for sexual integrity, I encourage you to dispel these myths in your mind with the truth from God's Word.

MYTH 1: There's nothing wrong with comparing myself or my husband to other people.

TRUTH: "When they measure themselves by themselves and compare themselves with themselves, they are not wise." (2 Corinthians 10:12)

MYTH 2: I am mature enough to watch any movie or television show, read any book, listen to any music, or surf any Web sites without being affected in any way.

TRUTH: "The good [woman] brings good things out of the good stored up in [her] heart, and the evil [woman] brings evil things out of the evil stored up in [her] heart." (Luke 6:45)

MYTHS 3 and 4: It doesn't hurt anyone if I fantasize about someone other than my husband when we make love, and thinking about what kind of man I'd like to have if my husband were to die is not a big deal, as long as I am not plotting how to carry that out!

TRUTH: "Those who live according to the sinful nature have their minds set on what that nature desires; but those who live in accordance with the Spirit have their minds set on what the Spirit desires. The mind of sinful man is death, but the mind controlled by the Spirit is life and peace; the sinful mind is hostile to God. It does not submit to God's law, nor can it do so. Those controlled by the sinful nature cannot please God. You, however, are controlled not by the sinful nature but by the Spirit, if the Spirit of God lives in you." (Romans 8:5-9)

MYTH 5: Masturbation does not hurt me, my relationship with my (current or future) husband, or my relationship with God.

TRUTH: "It is God's will that you should be sanctified: that you should avoid sexual immorality; that each of you should learn to control [her] own body in a way that is holy and honorable, not in passionate lust like the heathen, who do not know God." (1 Thessalonians 4:3-5)

MYTH 6: Because I feel so sexually tempted, I must already be guilty, so why bother resisting?

TRUTH: "For we do not have a high priest who is unable to sympathize with our weaknesses, but we have one who has been tempted in every way, just as we are—yet was without sin. Let us then approach the throne of grace with confidence, so that we may receive mercy and find grace to help us in our time of need." (Hebrews 4:15-16)

MYTH 7: There's no one who would really understand my struggle.

TRUTH: "No temptation has seized you except what is common to [woman]. And God is faithful; he will not let you be tempted beyond what you can bear. But when you are tempted, he will also provide a way out so that you can stand up under it." (1 Corinthians 10:13)

Jesus said, "If you hold to my teaching, you are really my disciples. Then you will know the truth, and the truth will set you free."

—John 8:31-32

time for a new revolution

Do not conform any longer to the pattern of this world, but be transformed by the renewing of your mind. Then you will be able to test
and approve what God's will is—his good, pleasing and perfect will.

ROMANS 12:2

When I recall my preteen years, my eagerness to speed through puberty stands out
in my mind. Tired of being treated like a little girl, I wanted so desperately to grow
up and become a woman, so I began practicing for the part. I took notice of how
modern women dressed, walked, talked, and acted and tried to mimic their performance. During this phase in the 1970s, the Enjoli perfume commercial aired on
our television repeatedly. A beautiful blonde in a form-fitting red dress fanned a
fistful of dollar bills, twirled a frying pan in the air, then threw herself into a man's
lap and seductively ran her fingers through his hair. The sultry words she wailed
were, "I'm a WOMAN!"

As Hollywood painted the picture of the liberated woman, most of us were
making mental notes and preparing to waltz blindly into Satan's trap. Don't get me
wrong; I'm thrilled that the women's liberation movement brought us freedom to
vote, get an education, and find satisfaction in careers. But the power plays, quests
for control, and manipulation games that have come with it have often buried
women up to their necks in the ashes of burned bras.

Since this liberation movement, women have been bombarded with messages
that we must be in shape, in love, and in control and that being sexy is of utmost
priority. With television, music, movies, magazines, romance novels, and the Internet, nothing short of living under a rock will keep women's minds from being

whirled by the world. But when did this sexual revolution begin, and how have we managed to come this far?

A JOURNEY THROUGH TIME

If we looked to American history books for clues, we'd see that in the early 1900s burlesque theaters opened with lewd jokes, skits, and songs; suggestive dancing; and near-nude female performers. Buxom beauty Mae West got her start in show business by entertaining the crowds at such theaters. By the 1920s the striptease had become the featured act in most of these shows. According to the *New Standard Encyclopedia,* "Burlesque disappeared completely in the 1960s. It had come to seem old-fashioned and rather tame compared to the sexual explicitness and salacious humor that had developed in nightclubs and motion pictures."[1]

Coming out of World War II, women were hungry for lighthearted entertainment and star-struck fans attempted to embrace (literally!) such suave celebrities as Frank Sinatra, Bing Crosby, and Rock Hudson with reckless abandon. Female sex symbols of this era were voluptuous women—Jane Russell, Jayne Mansfield, and Betty Grable. And who can ever forget Marilyn Monroe, whose personal life produced three failed marriages, multiple affairs, and several attempts at suicide, the last of which would take her life but not her sex-kitten legacy?

In the 1960s, the invasion of the Beatles singing "Revolution" birthed a greater awareness of the cultural shift in our country. Wearing Elvis's "Blue Suede Shoes," we gyrated toward sexual liberty and rebellion against authority at breakneck speeds. In the 1970s hippies began shouting, "Make love not war!" and "If it feels good, do it!" became the standard that governed sexual conduct. With the debut of *Charlie's Angels* and *10,* hairdressers and fitness centers made a fortune from the number of Farrah Fawcett and Bo Derek wannabes. Robert Palmer summarized the epidemic of the 1980s with his song, "Addicted to Love!" and even though Madonna was singing, "Like a Virgin," she wasn't teaching women to dress and act like one. The '90s will go down in history as the decade that Britney Spears graduated from her Mickey Mouseketeer hat into leather halter tops and hip-hugger jeans. Now in the twenty-first century, the sexual messages are so numerous that the downward spiral seems to be a big blur.

What kinds of things are being communicated to us by society today? I walk through the mall and hope that my daughter can avoid being influenced by the huge display in the Abercrombie & Fitch window—a picture of two girls and a guy in bed together—or the Victoria's Secret display or the Frederick's of Hollywood display. Even some of the displays in the JC Penney aisles have become extremely erotic. I drive through downtown Dallas and can't help but notice the frequent appearance of scantily clad women on billboards, usually for alcohol or "gentlemen's clubs" (although you'd never meet a gentleman there). I walk through a bookstore, and a graphic cover touting *The Joy of Gay Sex* catches my eye. No wonder there are men and women turning to sex outside of marriage (with members of the opposite and of the same sex). It's what society tries to convince us is desirable and acceptable. I rarely see advertisements depicting good, clean, healthy, fun sex *within a monogamous marriage relationship.*

Things have certainly changed. One hundred years ago Christians were upset over the private burlesque shows that traveled from town to town. Today young Christian women stroll down the street with pierced belly buttons glaring below skin-tight cropped tops, completely unaware of the effect they are having on men (or maybe they are aware). In 1939, *Gone with the Wind* brought gasps as Clark Gable's famous shocking line, "I don't give a ——!" made headline news. Today, moviemakers intentionally add vulgarity and sexual scenes to their movie just to attract more viewers with a PG-13 or R rating. Pornographic magazines once had to be sought out, found only on the highest bookracks in plain, brown wrappers and sold only to mature patrons. Today if you are old enough to know how to surf the Net, you can usher unlimited pornographic material into your own home via the click of a mouse.

However, the epidemic of sexual immorality began long before pornography or the burlesque shows of the early 1900s. Since the very beginning of time, Satan has used sex to create a cultural climate that lures us away from the holiness God calls us to. The book of Genesis reports the distortion of sexuality in seven different ways: polygamy (4:19), homosexuality (19:5), fornication and rape (34:2), prostitution (38:15), incest (38:16-18), and evil seduction (39:7). Sexuality has been one of Satan's favorite tools to cause believers confusion and moral failure ever since then. A trip back to the Garden of Eden will help us to understand how we've given Satan free reign in this world to create such a cultural climate.

THE GIFT EVE GAVE AWAY

In the first chapter of Genesis, we see that God created man and woman in His image and placed them in the Garden of Eden with the intention of having them rule and reign over everything. To visualize this picture, imagine God's giving Adam and Eve a beautifully wrapped gift box. Inside is a gift called *authority.* God gave this gift of authority to Adam and Eve, intending them to act wisely as stewards over all creation.

But the crafty serpent, perhaps knowing that the woman is enticed by what she hears, hissed in Eve's ear something about how she could have the power of God's wisdom if she took a bite of the forbidden fruit. Because Eve had been given authority to rule and reign over this creature, not the other way around, her response should have been to shut him up and send him packing when he tried to tempt her into disobeying God. But mesmerized by the enticement of power, Eve sank her teeth into the forbidden fruit, making the most bitter mistake of her life, a mistake which resulted in her being the one to have to pack up and leave paradise forever. Her sin was rebellion against her Creator, but the underlying tragedy was that she gave away her gift of authority to the crafty serpent.

Once sin entered into the hearts of humans, they no longer possessed the authority to rule and reign in the world. They gave that gift to Satan when they rebelled against God. That is when Satan became the ruler of this world, simply because humanity gave him the authority.

Previously Adam and Eve had been at perfect peace in their relationship with God and with each other, but the transfer of this gift from their hands into Satan's brought all that to an end. They once felt acceptance but now felt rejection. Their sense of belonging turned to loneliness and their feelings of competence gave way to feelings of inadequacy. Their sense of identity turned to confusion and their security faded into anxiety. Whereas they once felt significance, they now felt worthlessness. Their perfect relationship with God dwindled into a spiritual void.

The devil knew he now possessed this gift, and so did God. Satan actually flaunted his authority in front of Jesus' face, daring Him to try to take it back by playing Satan's twisted game rather than submitting to God's plan of restoring the gift of authority to humankind (a plan that would require the shedding of His blood unto death). Luke 4:5-7 says, "The devil led [Jesus] up to a high place and showed him in an instant all the kingdoms of the world. And he said to him, 'I will give you all their authority and splendor, for it has been given to me, and I can give it to anyone I want to. So if you worship me, it will be all yours.'"

Jesus answered Satan, "It is written: 'Worship the Lord your God and serve him only'" (Luke 4:8). Notice that Jesus didn't deny the devil's *current* authority over the kingdoms of the earth. But He knew what the future held and that it was just a matter of time before that authority would change hands and be returned to the rightful owner. He knew that He could never sin and win that authority back, therefore Jesus chose God's plan to restore and entrust that authority to humanity once again through His death and resurrection and the coming of the Holy Spirit.

Let's go back to the garden scene (Genesis 3) to see how the story unfolded. God's sovereign justice required consequences for humanity's deliberate disobedience. First, God cursed the serpent and promised that the woman's offspring would crush his head (a promise that was fulfilled with Christ's victory over Satan). Then God promised to increase Eve's pains in childbearing and said, "Your desire

Adam and Eve Created in His Image (Genesis 1 and 2)	Adam and Eve Chose to Try to Be Like God (Genesis 3)	This Rebellion Resulted in Pain (Genesis 3 and 4)
Acceptance	Sin	Rejection
Belonging		Loneliness
Competence		Inadequacy
Equity		Exploitation
Identity		Confusion
Security		Anxiety
Significance		Worthlessness
Transcendence		Spiritual Void

Figure 4.1: Expelled from Eden[2]

will be for your husband, and he will rule over you" (verse 16). Then He punished Adam by cursing the ground and requiring that man work diligently to make the earth produce food (verses 17-19).

But let's rewind back to verse 16. When God told Eve, "Your desire will be for your husband, and he will rule over you," was He saying that women will have a *sexual* desire for their husbands? While most scholars read the first half of this sentence and make that assumption, I want to challenge you to look at the entire sentence before drawing your conclusion. It says, "Your desire will be for your husband, *and* he will *rule* over you."

Why would Scripture use these two phrases in the same sentence? Could they perhaps be connected? I think they are. I believe a woman's *desire* and the issue of *rulership* or *power* are related in a way that unwraps some of the mystery behind a woman's sexual conduct (or misconduct, rather). I believe that the desire for power (and the belief that men possess the power women crave) is what causes many women to seduce men, as well as what prompts some to use sex as a bargaining tool in their marriage. It's not as much sex or love that these women are in pursuit of as it is the power behind bringing a man to his knees with her charms.

When we discovered as young women that our curvaceous bodies or pretty faces would turn heads, it awakened us to a form of power that we may have never known as preadolescent girls. For some of us, that power was intoxicating…perhaps even addicting. Turning the head of a peer became a small thrill, while turning the head of an older, important man held huge payoffs for our egos. Whether it was the captain of the football team, the college professor, or the head of the department at work, sharing in the power of important people by aligning ourselves with them in relationship gave us a distorted sense of significance.

When men resist allowing a woman to share in their power or rob them of their personal resolve, some women have been known to become quite manipulative, using sexual prowess or emotional entanglements in order to firmly establish or hold on to their sense of power. Unfortunately, even victory in these manipulation games leaves us power-*hungry* and *powerless* over our fleshly desires.

If you want to know how to satisfy your hunger for power (which is a normal part of the human condition but can certainly drive you much further into this battle than you want to go), I'll let you in on a secret: The sense of power that will satisfy your soul is not found in *men.* It is found only in *God.* Does God give His power to men? Yes. But do you need to go through a man to receive God's power? No. The only middleman you need to tap into God's power is the Holy Spirit. And when you discover the power of the Holy Spirit to help you live an abundantly fulfilled life, you will know that seductive power pales in comparison.

THE PURSUIT OF POWER AND LONGING FOR LOVE

Most of my single days are a tragic testimony of a young woman striving to gain some sense of power through inappropriate relationships with men. Rather than use what beauty God had given me to bring glory to Him, I used it as bait to lure men into feeding my ego. Rather than inspiring men to worship God, I subconsciously wanted them to worship me, and if I was successful in hooking a man with my charms, I secretly felt powerful.

I never realized these tragic truths until I went through counseling after I was married. I was seeking to understand why I still felt tempted outside of my marriage, so my therapist asked me to spend a week making a list of every man I had ever been with sexually or had pursued emotionally. I was shocked and saddened to see how long my list had grown through the years.

At the next visit, she asked me to spend a week praying and asking myself, "What do each of these men have in common?" God showed me that each relationship had been with someone who was older than I and in some form of authority over me—my professor, my boss, my lawyer.

As I searched my soul to discern why such a common thread existed in my relational pursuits, the root of the issue became evident: my hunger for power over a man. Due to my feelings of powerlessness in my relationship with an authoritarian father, I had subconsciously been re-creating authoritative relationships in order to "win this time." Each time I got the upper hand in a relationship, subconsciously seducing my prey into catering to my needs and desires, it was really as if I were saying, "See Dad! Someone does love me! I *am* worthy of attention and affection!"

In my attempts to fill the father-shaped hole in my heart and establish some semblance of self-worth through these dysfunctional relationships, I was creating a long list of shameful liaisons and a trunk load of emotional baggage. I was overlooking the only true source of satisfaction and self-worth: an intimate relationship with my heavenly Father. Through pursuing this relationship first and foremost, not only has Jesus become my first love and given me a sense of worth beyond what any man could give, He has also restored my relationship with my earthly father and helped me remain faithful to my husband. (We'll talk more about this intimate relationship with our heavenly Father in chapter 11.)

I believe that many women who struggle with sexual and/or emotional integrity are still little girls trapped in a grown woman's body, desperately seeking a father figure to give them the love they craved as a child. This pursuit of "love" takes the form of searching for intimacy and closeness, and unfortunately the world we live in teaches that this intimacy and closeness can be found only through sexual relationships. However, as many women have painfully discovered, relationships can be built entirely on sex and still be devoid of any intimacy or closeness at all, which leaves us feeling even more powerless to have our needs met.

Unfortunately, women have long been using sex in order to get their own needs met. In fact, this has been going on since biblical times. Paul preached against it in his first letter to Timothy when he wrote, "I do not permit a woman to teach or to have authority over a man; she must be silent" (2:12). Some people have interpreted this verse as an injunction to keep women from any form of leadership in the church, but I believe it has nothing to do with teaching the gospel or justly exercising her authority to lead others to Christ. As I've researched the actual Greek word that Paul was using for "authority," I have come to believe he was addressing the exact issue we're talking about in this chapter: *women using sex to exert power over men.*

The word Paul used for "authority" is the Greek word *authentein,* and not all scholars agree on its meaning. Some have translated it as "to usurp authority, domineer, or exercise authority over," but others translate it as "to involve someone in soliciting sexual liaisons." In other words, the verse could be read, "I do not permit a woman to teach sexual immorality or to involve a man in sexual sin."[3]

Here are a few other examples of women who are guilty of manipulation games in their quest to gain a sense of power over men:

- Corin confesses that when she dresses in the morning, she considers what men she will be meeting with that day and chooses her attire based on whether she will need to sway a man's decision in a business matter. (Corin is abusing her power by using her sex appeal to manipulate men into giving her what she wants.)

- Trina has little interest in Kurt, a male coworker who obviously thinks the world of her, the way he heaps compliments on her. However, she will go out to lunch with Kurt if he offers to buy or if she just needs an ego boost. (Trina is taking advantage of Kurt's affection and his pocketbook with no intention of ever reciprocating his feelings.)

- Vicki admits that when she overspends the budget, she often initiates sex with her husband before breaking the news to him. (Vicki uses sex to soften the blow of money mismanagement.)

- A recent divorcée, Deborah has reentered the dating scene. She finds that when a man responds to her advances for emotional connection, she eventually loses interest. However, if he plays hard to get, she can't get him out of her mind. She thrives on the challenge of conquering a man's resolve. (Deborah isn't as interested in a genuine, intimate relationship as she is boosting her own ego by turning a man's head and luring him in with her seductive power.)

- Every Sunday morning Jennifer dresses her best and scans the crowd throughout the church service to see who is stealing a glance at her. (In Jennifer's heart, going to church is more about getting the worship she longs to receive herself rather than offering worship to God.)

A MOVEMENT THAT HAS MOVED TOO FAR

"Men's Top 10 Sex Wants"[4]
"The Secret Sex Move He's Got to Feel to Believe"[5]
"The #1 Thing He Craves in Bed"[6]

These are just three of many similar magazine headlines at the grocery store checkout counter. The numerous articles on topics like these indicate that many women today want sexual prowess, power, and creative ways to manipulate men into doing what they want. The headlines of local newspapers point to a sex-saturated culture, as do safe-sex programs in public schools, pro-choice rallies promoting legalized abortion, and gay and lesbian rights activists marching for their cause.

What started over a hundred years ago as a women's movement for equal rights, equal pay, and equal opportunity has evolved into something it was never intended to be. We are living in an age where many women are actually more promiscuous than men. Now women are trying to exert power over others, insisting on their rights to make "choices" while (1) disregarding respect for men's rights to avoid sexual temptations and (2) disregarding God's design for sex to create life and to bring intimacy between a husband and a wife.

Diane Passno explains in her book *Feminism: Mystique or Mistake?* that what actually started out as a Christian effort to rid society of the negative effects of alcoholism (the temperance movement) and to gain equal rights for women has evolved into a movement that has moved too far away from its roots.

> I have felt a keen disappointment in the feminists of my generation, whose main message has been one of embracing reproductive freedom [abortion], the lesbian lifestyle, and a self-centered "victim" philosophy that is not only tiresome, but self-defeating. [National Organization for Women (NOW)] claims a membership of one-half million, representing less than one-half of 1 percent of women in the United States today.... The majority of women in this country do not align themselves with the message or the angry, brow-beating, outspoken women who deliver it. The feminists of the earlier half of the century who fought for the rights of women to vote and to hold equal employment won battles that needed to be fought...battles about which all women could agree and could be like-minded combatants. However, the feminists of the current generation have an agenda that is very divisive in nature, and the majority of women simply are not getting on the bandwagon and yelling "tallyho" to support it....
>
> How did a social movement that began under the title of the Women's Christian Temperance Union, founded by Christian women grounded in Scripture, get so mangled 100 years later? How did a women's movement that preached social justice, established on Christian principles, become a movement that mocks those same principles today? How could a movement

that stressed moral purity for both sexes become a movement that preaches sexual freedom with no restraint, lesbian rights, and a hatred for the male gender?[7]

As a result of this movement gone awry, many women no longer govern themselves by what is absolutely true (according to Scripture); instead they govern themselves by what is absolutely popular. I call it Popular Morality, which says, "If everybody else is doing it, so can I." But let's remember what our mothers used to tell us: "If everybody else jumped off a building, would you do it?" She was right. Not everybody is doing it (*it* could be anything—sex outside of marriage, abortion, lesbianism, fantasy, masturbation, and so on), and even if they are, that doesn't make it the right or smart thing to do.

TIME FOR A NEW REVOLUTION

Sociologist and historian Carle Zimmerman wrote a book titled *Family and Civilization* based on his observations that the disintegration of various cultures directly paralleled the decline of family life in those cultures. The eight common threads that Zimmerman identified as running throughout each documented civilization that has come to ruin thus far include:

1. Marriage loses its sacredness and divorce becomes common.
2. The traditional meaning of the marriage ceremony is lost.
3. Feminist movements abound.
4. Public disrespect for parents and authority increase.
5. Juvenile delinquency, promiscuity, and rebellion accelerate.
6. People with traditional marriages refuse to accept family responsibilities.
7. Desire for and acceptance of adultery grow.
8. Interest in sexual perversions and sex-related crimes increase.[8]

While you may think that, based on the current ills of our society, Zimmerman wrote this book recently, he actually published this work in 1947. Do these common threads also run throughout our society today? You be the judge.

- Approximately 50 percent of marriages end in divorce.
- Sixty-five percent of children will grow up fatherless for a time in their lives.

- Almost 50 percent of women are raped by someone they know before they turn eighteen.
- Cohabitation is at an all-time high, and 95 percent of couples say they do not want a marriage like the one their parents had.[9]

These statistics make me wonder how much longer it will be before our civilization comes to ruin as well. I believe it is time for a new cultural revolution—one where we reclaim and exercise our authority over all of creation (including Satan). Once we reclaim this authority and stop submitting ourselves to a culture that is leading us astray, we can discover new levels of sexual integrity, enjoy genuine intimacy in marriage, and experience the satisfaction of our innermost desires through righteous relationships.

RECLAIMING THE GIFT OF AUTHORITY

Turning the tide in our culture may seem like an impossible task, but we are not alone in this challenge. *God* will turn the tide *through* us. He simply asks us to submit our own lives to Him and to be a witness to what His power and love can do. As more and more women receive this revelation and share this wisdom with

I AM ACCEPTED IN CHRIST
• I am God's child (John 1:12).
• I am Christ's friend (John 15:15).
• I have been justified (Romans 5:1).
• I am united with the Lord and one with him in spirit (1 Corinthians 6:17).
• I have been bought at a price; I belong to God (1 Corinthians 6:20).
• I am a member of Christ's body (1 Corinthians 12:27).
• I am a saint (Ephesians 1:1).
• I have been adopted as God's child (Ephesians 1:5).
• I have direct access to God through the Holy Spirit (Ephesians 2:18).
• I have been redeemed and forgiven of all my sins (Colossians 1:14).
• I am complete in Christ (Colossians 2:10).

Figure 4.2: Who I Am in Christ[10]   *(continued on next two pages)*

others, the tide will eventually turn on its own. We need to begin by focusing on our own behaviors so that we no longer allow the world to influence us. This can only be done by personally reclaiming the gift of authority that Eve originally gave away.

In order to reclaim this gift, we must realize that God is the only true source of power. The only way to experience the power we crave is to connect intimately with Him. When we do, He meets our innermost needs for love, acceptance, and significance. This results in the power to exert self-control. God promises to give us self-control, along with many other attributes, when we allow ourselves to be led by the Holy Spirit. "But the fruit of the Spirit is love, joy, peace, patience, kindness, goodness, faithfulness, gentleness and self-control" (Galatians 5:22-23).

Once we connect to the ultimate source of power and discover the true power of self-control, we can take back the authority that Eve once gave to Satan. First John 4:4 reminds us that greater is He who is in you (Holy Spirit) than he who is in the world (Satan).

How exactly do we take this authority back? By understanding who we really are as a result of Christ's dying to set us free from the laws of sin and death. How

I Am Secure in Christ
• I am free forever from condemnation (Romans 8:1-2).
• I am assured that all things work together for good (Romans 8:28).
• I am free from any condemning charges against me (Romans 8:33-34).
• I cannot be separated from the love of God (Romans 8:35, 38-39).
• I have been established, anointed, and sealed by God (2 Corinthians 1:21-22).
• I am confident that the good work God has begun in me will be perfected (Philippians 1:6).
• I am a citizen of heaven (Philippians 3:20).
• I am hidden with Christ in God (Colossians 3:3).
• I have not been given a spirit of fear, but of power, love, and self-discipline (2 Timothy 1:7).
• I can find grace and mercy to help me in time of need (Hebrews 4:16).
• I am born of God, and the evil one cannot touch me (1 John 5:18).

Figure 4.2: Who I Am in Christ[10]

(continued)

we see ourselves affects how we live and the decisions we make. If we see ourselves as weak, tempted beyond control, or needy, then that is how we will behave. But if that is what we still believe and how we still behave, then Christ's death on the cross was in vain. He died so that His Holy Spirit could fill our emptiness, heal our hurts, and satisfy our every need.

Sadly, most believers do not understand who they really are, who God made them to be, the authority He intended them to possess, or how Christ can meet their innermost desires for acceptance, security, and significance. In his book *Living Free in Christ,* Neil T. Anderson summarizes who we are as a result of what Christ did for us and how we possess all power and authority simply as a result of our relationship with God. (Please see Figure 4.2, starting on page 61.)

THE THIRTY-DAY CHALLENGE

When I speak I often challenge women to avoid any television, movies, books, magazines, or music that would influence their thinking about themselves or about men in a negative way for thirty days. Copy the scriptures from Figure 4.2, tape

I AM SIGNIFICANT IN CHRIST
• I am the salt and light of the earth (Matthew 5:13-14).
• I am a branch of the true vine, a channel of his life (John 15:1,5).
• I have been chosen and appointed to bear fruit (John 15:16).
• I am a personal witness of Christ (Acts 1:8).
• I am God's temple (1 Corinthians 3:16).
• I am a minister of reconciliation (2 Corinthians 5:17-20).
• I am God's coworker (2 Corinthians 6:1).
• I am seated with Christ in the heavenly realms (Ephesians 2:6).
• I am God's workmanship (Ephesians 2:10).
• I may approach God with freedom and confidence (Ephesians 3:12).
• I can do all things through Christ who gives me strength (Philippians 4:13).

Figure 4.2: Who I Am in Christ[10]

them onto your bathroom mirror, and repeat them aloud to yourself every morning for each of those thirty days. Repeat the exercise whenever you begin to feel insecure, lonely, or tempted to manipulate someone else into meeting your needs.

Getting to know God more intimately means, in part, learning how He feels about you and understanding the provisions He has made in order to satisfy your innermost desires to feel loved, needed, and powerful (a righteous form of power, not a manipulative one). This is a great way to discover who you really are—not as the world tries to program you to be, but as your Maker designed you to be. Once you allow God to correct your beliefs about yourself, those beliefs will begin driving your decisions, your behaviors will follow directly behind, and you will have victory in this battle against sexual compromise.

> *The world doesn't fight fair. But we don't live or fight our battles that way.... The tools of our trade aren't for marketing or manipulation, but they are for demolishing that entire massively corrupt culture. We use our powerful God-tools for smashing warped philosophies, tearing down barriers erected against the truth of God, fitting every loose thought and emotion and impulse into the structure of life shaped by Christ. Our tools are ready at hand for clearing the ground of every obstruction and building lives of obedience into maturity.*
>
> —*2 Corinthians 10:3-5* (MSG)

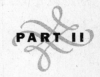

designing
a new defense

taking thoughts captive

> For though we live in the world, we do not wage war as the world does.
> The weapons we fight with are not weapons of the world.... We take
> captive every thought to make it obedient to Christ.
>
> 2 CORINTHIANS 10:3-5

You are getting into a four-door car by yourself. It's late at night and you are in a rough neighborhood. In order to feel safe, what is the first thing you are going to do when you get in the car? Right. Lock the doors.

How many doors will you lock? You may think this is a silly question, but think about it. If you only locked one or two or even three of the doors, would you be safe? Of course not. All four doors must be locked to keep out an unwelcome intruder.

The same is true with keeping out unwelcome sexual temptations. These temptations can invade our lives and eventually give birth to sin in four ways. The thoughts we choose to entertain in our minds can influence us. The words we speak or the conversations we engage in can lure us down unrighteous, dangerous paths. So can the failure to guard our hearts from getting involved in unhealthy relationships. And when we allow our bodies to be in the wrong place at the wrong time with the wrong person, we can be led toward sexual compromise.

Even if we leave only one of these doors unlocked, we are vulnerable. We must guard all four areas (our minds, our hearts, our mouths, and our bodies) to have any hope of remaining safe and maintaining sexual integrity. We'll discuss the first of these areas in this chapter and the other areas in each of the next three chapters.

WHAT'S ON YOUR MIND?

In the movie *What Women Want,* Nick Marshall (Mel Gibson) develops a tele-pathic ability to hear each thought, opinion, and desire that goes through every woman's head.

Imagine this: Tomorrow morning you wake up and every man on the planet has developed the ability to read your mind just by being in your presence. Does the thought make you nervous? You bet it does! Especially when we consider the thoughts that roll around in our minds on a regular basis that we would never articulate to anyone! Thoughts such as:

- *I wonder if he thinks I'm attractive?*
- *I wonder if he knows that I think he's attractive?*
- *I wonder what it would be like to kiss him?*
- *Could he be The One?*

And what if every woman developed this ability too? They might hear things such as:

- *She really thinks she's something, doesn't she?*
- *How did she get a handsome guy like that?*
- *I wonder if her husband would be interested in me if anything ever happened to her?*
- *At least I'm not that fat!*

Even though we can rest assured that men and women aren't likely to develop this sensitivity any time soon, we have an even bigger concern. God has had this ability all along. Could you, like David, be so bold as to pray such a thing as this: "Test me, O LORD, and try me, examine my heart and my mind" (Psalm 26:2)?

Notice David didn't say, "Examine my actions." He asked God to examine what was inside of him. What about you? What's on the inside of your heart and mind? Even women who have never had a serious relationship nor been involved in inappropriate sexual activity often have impure thoughts and longings. Regard-less of our past, all of us share in this struggle.

But just because all women have tempting thoughts, it doesn't mean that it is wise to indulge in them or entertain them. It's one thing to have random sexual thoughts or inappropriate emotional longings. We are only human. God does not hold these things against us. It is another, more dangerous thing to entertain these thoughts in our minds over and over or to indulge in frequent fantasies with little regard to the nature of what is going on in our heads. As the famous quote says,

> Sow a thought, reap an action;
> Sow an action, reap a habit;
> Sow a habit, reap a character;
> Sow a character, reap a destiny.
> —Samuel Smiles

I want the thoughts that I sow to reap positive actions and habits so that I can have Christlike character and fulfill the destiny God has for me. I'm sure you want the same, so let's examine three questions about our thought life:

- What thoughts does God say are appropriate or inappropriate?
- What effect do our thoughts have on this battle for sexual and emotional integrity?
- How can we guard our minds against influences that cause us to sin?

KEEPING THE MAIN THING THE MAIN THING

Do you recall what Jesus said is by far the most important thing in life?

> "Love the Lord your God with all your heart and with all your soul and with all your mind." This is the first and greatest commandment. (Matthew 22:37-38)

This verse doesn't say that Jesus wants us to love the Lord with whatever is left of our heart, soul, and mind. Nor does it say that God should consume our every thought every minute of the day. Most of us can't sit around all day and meditate on God. He knows you have a life. He's the one who gave it to you, and He wants you to be a good steward over your marriage relationship, your children's education, your career, your household responsibilities, your church and social commitments, and so on.

According to these verses, Jesus wants us to love God *more* than any of the other things that demand our time and attention. We are to love God above anything else in this world, with as much strength and passion as each of us possibly can. We demonstrate this love for God by focusing our thoughts and energies on those things He's prepared for us to do and that are also pleasing to Him. God wants us to do just as Paul encouraged the people of Philippi to do:

> Whatever is true, whatever is noble, whatever is right, whatever is pure,
> whatever is lovely, whatever is admirable—if anything is excellent or praise-
> worthy—think about such things. (Philippians 4:8)

To show you how this works, I'll tell you about a typical day in my life when I'm able to keep my focus on godly things. I usually wake up with a worship song rolling around in my head, and I'll more than likely hum a few bars or even bellow it out in the shower. As I prepare for the day, I try to look my best to give a positive impression to the people I will encounter. As I make breakfast, get the kids ready for school, make a grocery list, fill the car up with gas, and drop bills by the post office, I am serving my family. As I go about my work responsibilities, I do it for the sake of advancing God's kingdom. As I send a note to a hurting coworker, forward a funny e-mail to my friend, call to check on my neighbor, I do it to build and maintain healthy and positive relationships. All of these thoughts and actions are acts of responsible stewardship. I do them out of appreciation for the family and friends that God has given me. Is God my one and only constant thought throughout the day? No. But even as I think on the various other things that demand my attention, am I loving God with all my heart, soul, and mind? Absolutely. When we demonstrate responsible stewardship of the life He has given us, our lives offer proof of our love.

BACK TO THE BIBLE

The only reliable standard we can use to measure our thoughts to determine if they are appropriate or inappropriate is God's Word. Hebrews 4:12-13 says:

For the word of God is living and active. Sharper than any double-edged sword, it penetrates even to dividing soul and spirit, joints and marrow; *it judges the thoughts* and attitudes of the heart. Nothing in all creation is hidden from God's sight. Everything is uncovered and laid bare before the eyes of him to whom we must give account. (emphasis added)

Before we can determine what sexual or romantic thoughts are unacceptable in God's eyes, however, it would be beneficial to know what sexual acts are forbidden in Scripture. In the process of writing their book *Intimate Issues,* Linda Dillow and Lorraine Pintus searched from Genesis to Revelation to discover everything that God has to say about sexual behaviors. According to their study, Scripture prohibits the following sexual acts:

1. *Fornication*—immoral sex, including intercourse outside of marriage
2. *Adultery*—sex with someone who is not your spouse (Jesus expanded this definition in Matthew 5:28 to include not just physical acts, but emotional and mental acts as well.)
3. *Homosexuality*—to engage in sexual practices with someone of the same sex
4. *Impurity*—to become defiled due to living out a secular or pagan lifestyle
5. *Orgies*—to engage in sex with more than one person at a time
6. *Prostitution*—receiving money in exchange for sexual acts
7. *Lustful passions*—unrestrained, indiscriminate sexual desire for men or women other than the person's marriage partner
8. *Sodomy*—sex between two males
9. *Obscenity and course jokes*—inappropriate sexual comments in a public setting
10. *Incest*—sex with family members[1]

For sexual acts not covered in this list, Dillow and Pintus recommend that women ask three questions to determine whether a particular sexual act is permissible. I recommend using the same questions to determine if particular thoughts are acceptable. These three questions include:

- *Is it prohibited in Scripture?* If not, we may assume it is permitted. "Everything is permissible for me" (1 Corinthians 6:12).

- *Is it beneficial?* Does the practice in any way harm the husband or wife or hinder the sexual relationship? If so, it should be rejected. "Everything is permissible for me—but not everything is beneficial" (1 Corinthians 6:12).

- *Does it involve anyone else?* Sexual activity is sanctioned by God for husband and wife only. If a sexual practice involves someone else or becomes public, it is wrong based on Hebrews 13:4, which warns us to keep the marriage bed undefiled.[2]

I conducted my own unofficial poll by asking a few women to tell me their most common fantasy or recurrent sexual thought. Here are some of their responses, as well as how these thoughts measure up using our three questions as a filter:

- Showering with my husband. Is it prohibited in Scripture? No. Is it beneficial? I'll bet her husband would think so. Does it involve anyone else? No. This is one thought that will enhance your sexual integrity, not compromise it.

- Having a romantic candlelit dinner with Richard Gere. Is it prohibited in Scripture? No. Is it beneficial? I can't imagine her husband would think so, nor does it make her feel more love for her husband. Does it involve anyone else? Yes. This is a thought that needs to be redirected to safer ground, such as having that same dinner with her husband instead.

- Having a threesome with my husband and another woman. Is it prohibited in Scripture? Yes. Is it beneficial? No. Does it involve anyone else? Yes. This is certainly dangerous thinking that needs to be avoided at every turn.

- Waking up in my husband's arms on a tropical vacation. Is it prohibited in Scripture? Certainly not. Is it beneficial? You bet. Does it involve anyone else? No. This dream is okay to hold on to.

We can use these questions as a filter for our thoughts or fantasies, as well as for anything else we expose our minds to (television, movies, books, magazines, chat rooms, and so on). Before I share some examples of how I have filtered these types of influences, let's look at how our thoughts can undermine our sexual and emotional integrity.

WEAKENING OUR DEFENSES

I watched a speaker bring several volunteers from the audience onstage in order to conduct an experiment about the power of our thoughts. He asked the group of individuals to think about the best thing in life that has ever happened to them. After a moment, he said, "Now that you have that thought planted firmly in your mind, I want you to put your arms straight out like you are making a cross with your body and hold your arms in this position, regardless of how hard I try to push them back down to your side."

The speaker appeared to be pretty strong, yet he could not overpower anyone's arms back down. He gave the volunteers a moment to recover, then said, "Now I want you to think about the worst thing in life that's ever happened to you, then assume the same position." One by one, the speaker effortlessly pushed their arms back down to their sides. His point was well-taken. Positive thoughts give us strength, while negative thoughts drain our strength.

In a similar way, our thoughts about our husbands (whether we think about him in a negative or positive light) and thoughts about inappropriate activities or relationships (whether we think about resisting such temptations or whether we entertain and envision ourselves engaged in these activities) can either strengthen or weaken our defense against sexual compromise.

I recall watching a movie many years back where a young man was fantasizing about a female stranger approaching him amorously, going straight for the kill by removing his black-rimmed glasses, running her fingers through his hair, embracing him firmly, and kissing him passionately. As young as I was when I witnessed this scene, I remember thinking, "Yeah, right. Dream on, buddy. Women don't operate like that."

A woman doesn't just walk up to a strange man, kiss him, and seduce him out of nowhere. But some women have done this very thing after they have known the man for some time and have entertained such thoughts in their heads over and over. Perhaps they've tested the water with a little flirting here and there to make sure he's responsive to their advances. Maybe they have even rehearsed the plan in order to make it foolproof. When a woman dwells on the possibility of engaging in this type of negative behavior, it can zap her strength to resist and cause her defenses to crumble.

Of course most women would never act out in such a blatant way. Whether the tighter reigns are a result of modesty, fear, disgust, or insecurity, many keep their affairs restricted to their minds. But when they allow their minds to envision being involved in an affair or in other inappropriate activities or relationships, they are paving the way for their defenses to become so weakened that they eventually act out their thoughts. Let me show you how this happens.

THINKING EQUALS REHEARSING

Imagine an actor preparing to perform in a play. She memorizes her lines, gets inside the character's head, and tries to imagine how this person would feel and act. She rehearses being that person. She thinks intently about doing what that person would do and saying what that person would say exactly the way she would say it. The more she's rehearsed being that character, the sharper and more "automatic" her performance.

Something similar happens when we fantasize sexually or emotionally about inappropriate or sinful behavior. We are rehearsing when we think about the conversations we would have with a particular man if we were ever alone with him, when we entertain thoughts of an intimate rendezvous, or wish that a certain man would take special notice of us. When we rehearse these scenarios, we imagine what we'll say and do in these encounters. Then when Satan lays the trap and leads that man your direction, guess what? We are more than likely going to play the part exactly the way we have rehearsed it. When we don't guard our minds in our relationships with men, we weaken our resistance before any encounter takes place.

But we do have some choice in the matter. We don't have to be sitting ducks. We can train our minds to mind.

TRAINING OUR MINDS TO MIND

One of my favorite sayings is: "You can't keep a bird from flying over your head, but you can keep him from building a nest in your hair!"

Even though inappropriate thoughts inevitably pop up into every person's mind, we do not have to entertain them. Such thoughts are not sin, but dwelling on such thoughts is essentially rehearsing for rebellion, and acting on such thoughts is sin. We can't keep from being tempted, but we can avoid rehearsing, and we can certainly refuse to sin. No temptation becomes sin without our permission.

So how do we keep the bird from building a nest in our hair? How do we avoid dwelling on random thoughts to the point that we are "rehearsing" rather than "rebuking" them? There are three primary ways, and I call them the Three Rs:

- Resisting
- Redirecting
- Renewing

RESISTING TEMPTATION AT THE GATE

Allowing your mind to be filled with images of sexually immoral or inappropriate behavior is like filling your mind with garbage. Garbage eventually rots, putrefying the soul and infecting your life and the lives of those you are closest to. One of the primary ways to avoid inappropriate fantasies and sexual misconduct is to resist such images and thoughts by limiting their access to your minds. This will require close monitoring of your reading, viewing, and listening habits, but once you make a habit of censorship, it will become second nature.

The following is a list of personal convictions I have incorporated into my life about what I look at and listen to, along with explanations of why I've made these choices. (You'll recognize the three-question filter mentioned earlier.) These convictions give me freedom to enjoy life without subjecting myself to temptations that might prove overwhelming. I hope they will spur your thinking about the ways that you can guard your mind against temptation as well.

- I avoid looking at any form of pornography. I believe it is forbidden in Scripture according to number 4 on the *Intimate Issues* list of God's sexual prohibitions (Impurity). It does not benefit my sex life, and it involves someone else outside my marriage. I don't want to have my focus pulled away from my husband and on to a stranger.

- I limit my television viewing and avoid watching daytime or evening soap operas. They do not benefit me in any way and are a waste of my time. Scripture prohibits the illicit scenarios on these shows. (They usually involve sex outside of marriage.) If there is a television show that I know will be uplifting and supportive of my Christian values, I'll sit down to watch it. But once it's over, so is my viewing time. I get up and move on to something more productive and beneficial.

- I don't listen to secular music. I have a lot of sexual memories that are attached to particular songs from my past. When I am out in public, I occasionally hear a song that sends me back to a particular place, time, or relationship, evoking memories I'd much rather forget. Funny how music has the power to do that. That is why I switched over ten years ago from my regular radio station to one that plays nothing but Christian contemporary music. Now when I hear a Christian song from my past, it brings to mind where I was spiritually when I first heard it. These musical spiritual markers remind me of how far God has brought me. With the wide variety of quality music today, Christian music is every bit as entertaining (and much more edifying!) as anything on the secular market.

- I choose not to read romance novels. I consider steamy romance novels to be pornography for females. (The sexually graphic pictures are mental rather than visual, which is more alluring to women.) They often glamorize sex outside of marriage and can arouse us sexually. I am also careful about Christian romance novels if I find myself comparing my husband to the hero in the story and thinking about all the ways Greg doesn't measure up. I want to protect my marriage by resisting any thoughts that may evoke feelings of disillusionment and disappointment with reality.

- I'm also very selective about the women's magazines I pick up because so many of the messages aren't helpful to me. When I read pages and pages of advice on how to be skinnier and look at the pencil-thin models in their underwear, I feel dissatisfied and unhappy with my body. After looking at all of the smooth, tight abdomens scattered throughout the magazine, I can get pretty depressed just looking at myself in the mirror—let alone giving my husband the pleasure of watching me undress. But when I avoid comparing myself and appreciate the strong, healthy body God gave me, I feel much better about my figure and give myself more freely and joyfully to my husband.

If you want to become a woman of sexual and emotional integrity, I urge you to ask God to help you create your own list of ways you can guard your mind against sexual temptation. Examine what you allow to come into your mind—through magazines, books, movies, television, radio, and the Internet.

Ask yourself:

- Does this glamorize ideas or situations that oppose my Christian values?
- Is it uplifting to my spirit, and does it make me grateful for what God has given me, or does it make me depressed and dissatisfied?
- Does this cause me to think about things that build my character, or does it tear it down?

Don't allow things to enter your mind that can distract you from being devoted to Christ and the things He has called you to do. Paul warned the Corinthians about this possibility when he wrote:

I am jealous for you with a godly jealousy. I promised you to one husband, to Christ, so that I might present you as a pure virgin to him. But I am afraid that just as Eve was deceived by the serpent's cunning, your minds may somehow be led astray from your sincere and pure devotion to Christ. (2 Corinthians 11:2-3)

Paul wasn't worried that the Corinthians weren't thinking about God twenty-four hours a day, seven days a week. His worry was that the things they were spending time thinking about would lead them in the opposite direction from God. Do the things that you fill your mind with lead you *toward* God or in a direction *opposite* from God?

Be honest with yourself and with God. Only He knows what is best for you. Invite Him to shine His spotlight of truth into your heart and mind, showing you what you can do to make your mind more resistant even to being tempted in the first place.

In addition to screening what you allow into your mind, you can mentally rehearse righteous responses to temptations. For instance, anytime you have inappropriate thoughts about someone or suspect that he may be coming your direction, imagine that, rather than giving in and being swept away like a character in some romance novel, you actually spurn his advances. See yourself nipping his interest in the bud. Even practice what you would say in response to his move to communicate beyond a shadow of a doubt that you are not a woman to be toyed with or someone who is so emotionally needy that she clings to anyone who treats her affectionately.

Here are some examples of how women have practiced their righteous responses to sexual and emotional temptations so that they were able to play the part to perfection when the spotlight was on them:

- Jana finds her newly divorced neighbor very attractive but wants to be certain that nothing inappropriate ever takes place between them. She has had thoughts that he may come over someday when her husband isn't home. Rather than imagining what it would be like to engage in a private conversation with him, Jana rehearses her line of defense. "My husband gets home after 5 P.M. Why don't you come back then and we'll all chat?" is how she will respond if he should ever show up on her doorstep.

- When a handsome, single coworker asked to meet with her privately about some issues affecting the office staff, Donna could have entertained thoughts of being alone with him. But as an ethical professional and a woman of integrity, she has rehearsed such situations. To guard against any possibility of inappropriate behavior, Donna replies, "When you notify my secretary to schedule the appointment, have her reserve the conference room."

(Because of the windows all around this room, she could hear his complaints privately without the two of them being isolated from other people.)

- At the office where she works as a dental hygienist, there is an attractive patient who is overly friendly with Linda each time he comes in. She knows that she must keep him at bay and imagines how she will shut him down when he makes inappropriate comments. She was seeing him to the front desk one day after he had a filling replaced, and as expected, he made his move. He placed his hand to the side of his sore cheek and said, "My mother would always kiss me where it hurts," and leaned Linda's direction. Linda responded without hesitation, "Well, I'm not your mother. When you go home, maybe she'll kiss it for you."

Practice makes perfect. Rehearsing their lines of defense enabled these women to resist temptation at the gate. Practicing your line of resistance will give you victory in the face of temptation as well.

REDIRECTING TEMPTING THOUGHTS

No matter how well you try to prevent tempting thoughts from entering through the gate of your mind, some will still slip through. Life itself brings temptation. The day you stop experiencing temptation isn't the day you stop reading romance novels or watching R-rated movies or the day you put a wedding band on your finger or the day you fast and pray for twelve hours straight. The day you stop experiencing temptation is the day you die.

Temptation comes part and parcel with being human, and you are no exception to that rule. For instance, perhaps a handsome boss evokes thoughts of sitting on his lap to take dictation. Maybe a passionate speaker stirs your spirit and you think for a moment how intriguing it would be to pick his brain over a private lunch. Sometimes a charming friend may cause you to wish you had met him before you committed your life to someone else.

Again, you haven't sinned when these thoughts pop up in your mind; they are merely pesky temptations. Every person on the planet experiences those at times. As I mentioned earlier, Scripture tells us that Jesus was tempted. It also tells us that He was sinless.

For we do not have a high priest who is unable to sympathize with our weaknesses, but we have one who has been tempted in every way, just as we are—yet was without sin. Let us then approach the throne of grace with confidence, so that we may receive mercy and find grace to help us in our time of need. (Hebrews 4:15-16)

Jesus understands what it feels like to be tempted. He was human too. He underwent the kinds of temptations we experience, yet he did not succumb to any of them. Because we have the Holy Spirit living in us, we can have the same victory if we learn to resist temptation by redirecting our thoughts.

Maybe you think, *But you just said I can't choose what thoughts come into my mind.* You are right. You can't prevent your mind from thinking random, inappropriate thoughts. But you can avoid entertaining them or dwelling on them.

In fact, you do this all the time. For example, when you arrive at an all-you-can-eat buffet, you can choose not to think about the twenty pounds you are trying to lose long enough to satisfy both your appetite and your sweet tooth, can't you? You can distract yourself with a telephone call from a friend when you have a list of house chores a mile long. Do you avoid thinking about the dirty clothes piling up in the basement when an opportunity to go shopping for new ones presents itself? Of course you do. We constantly make choices either to dwell on or disregard thoughts. We can either entertain ideas or ignore them, and sexual temptations or emotional cravings are no exception.

So what do we do when we come face to face with temptation?

- Rather than eyeballing an attractive man (men are not the only ones who have to control their eyes sometimes, are they?), avoid the second look and simply say to yourself, "Thank you, Lord, for Your awesome creation!" Idolatry is turning your attention from the Creator to the creation. When you notice a beautiful creation, just give credit to the Creator and move on.
- Meditate on scriptures that you have memorized as a way to keep your focus where it needs to be. One of my favorites to help me overcome temptation is Revelation 3:21: "To [her] who overcomes, I will give the right to sit with me on my throne, just as I overcame and sat down with my Father on his throne."

- Sing a song in your mind that helps you resist temptation. Steven Curtis Chapman's "Run Away" and Susan Ashton's "Walk on By" are two songs I've kept on mental standby. They've saved my thought life from taking a downward turn many times through the years.

- Pray for his wife. If he doesn't have one, pray for the one he will have someday. Or pray for your husband or the one you will have someday. Remind yourself that entertaining romantic or sexual thoughts about this person is mental adultery, and thank God that with His help you are able to keep your heart and mind pure.

- Finally, as I've heard Elisabeth Elliot say on her radio show, *Gateway to Joy*, when you come face to face with temptation simply *do the next thing*. Were you on your way to your office when you encountered this fine specimen? Then do not tarry. Go to work. Were you heading to meet a girlfriend for lunch? Don't keep her waiting. Go. If you want to remain on the path toward righteousness, don't allow yourself to get side-tracked by a handsome man if this is a relationship you should not entertain.

What is your game plan for redirecting your tempting thoughts? How will you respond when that bird flies overhead? Will you shoo it away, or will you allow it to build a nest in your hair?

RENEWING YOUR MIND

Once you begin stopping temptations at the gate and practice redirecting tempting thoughts, you are ready to begin the process of renewing your mind, which basically means putting new things into your brain so that you have better things to think on and meditate over. This is critical to your battle plan if you want to become a woman of sexual and emotional integrity.

Paul speaks of this process in Romans 12:1-2:

Therefore, I urge you, [sisters], in view of God's mercy, to offer your bodies as living sacrifices, holy and pleasing to God—this is your spiritual act of worship. Do not conform any longer to the pattern of this world, but be transformed by the renewing of your mind. Then you will be able to test and approve what God's will is—his good, pleasing and perfect will.

We are not to use our bodies for the fulfillment of our own selfish desires; they are instruments through which God can do His mighty work. In order to prepare ourselves for this purpose, we must resist what the world tries to put in our minds and keep a fresh flow of godly messages coming in. That is how we will know what God wants to do through us, because then His still, small voice won't be drowned out by the blaring noise of an ungodly world.

Susan's e-mail is a classic example of how we can stop temptations at the gate, redirect our thoughts, and renew our minds:

When I was thirteen, I stumbled upon an adult movie channel while babysitting for some family friends. I knew watching it was wrong, but I felt so aroused by it I began masturbating to it and did so each time I babysat, once the children were in bed. The first time I tried masturbating at home without watching this channel, I was surprised that all I had to do was close my eyes to replay any scene I mentally selected. I had total recall.

By the time I left for college, my masturbation and fantasy habit was all-consuming. Without access to a graphic television channel, I stole some pornographic magazines and hid them underneath the carpet lining of the trunk of my car. At least once or twice each week, I would drive to a secluded place, get out my magazines, and masturbate in my car.

Even after I was married, I would bring out a couple of my favorite magazines and one video I kept hidden from my husband and masturbate while he was at work. This went on for a couple of years until I had my first child. As I was baby-proofing the house, taking special precautions to keep dangerous things out of reach, I was stricken with the idea that my child might one day find my secret hiding place. I prayed about it and asked God to give me two things: (1) a clear sign that I should get rid of these things, and (2) the strength to resist ever replacing them once they were gone.

The next day I was thumbing through my Bible and came across this scripture:

> You were taught, with regard to your former way of life, to put off your old self, which is being corrupted by its deceitful desires; to be made new in the attitude of your minds; and to put on the new self, created to be like God in true righteousness and holiness. (Ephesians 4:22-24)

That was my sign. I threw everything out and vowed not to indulge in self-gratification any longer. I usually indulged in this practice during my baby's daily naptime, so I had to create a new ritual. I began not just reading my Bible, but studying passages of Scripture and meditating on them. I started a journal and began writing what I sensed the Lord wanted to teach me. I would pray about things that I had never previously taken the time to pray about. I purchased some greeting cards and sent notes to individuals God laid on my heart during my prayer time. If I had any time left over, I would put on some soft worship music and do some stretching exercises or straighten the house. I couldn't believe how quickly the hours passed and how much I looked forward to and enjoyed this special time.

Susan discovered the secret to living the overcoming life: *Either sin will keep you from the Bible, or the Bible will keep you from sin.*

Of course, reading or even studying the Bible won't keep you from sin. (Just look at all the pastors who are Bible scholars yet have engaged in sexual sin.) We have to *internalize* and *apply* what the Bible says. To renew the mind means to bring fresh, living thoughts into our minds in addition to keeping old, decaying thoughts at bay. Even though it's not humanly possible to empty your mind of garbage, it is possible to crowd the garbage out by filling your mind with pure thoughts. Your mind can only concentrate on so many things at once, and the more you concentrate on wholesome thoughts, the more your unwholesome thoughts will have to take a backseat. Some things we can tap into to help us renew our minds are:

- scripture memory
- Christian-living books
- praise and worship music
- value-based television and movies
- devotional books
- Christian magazines
- prayer journals
- conversations with other Christians

Perhaps you can add to this list other ways to keep your mind full of godly messages that will help crowd out the sinful messages.

By resisting temptation at the gate, redirecting tempting thoughts, and renewing our minds we can develop an attitude such as David had when he asked, "Search me, O God, and know my heart; test me and know my anxious thoughts. See if there is any offensive way in me, and lead me in the way everlasting" (Psalm 139:23-24).

As you dive into the things of God and go deep in your spiritual walk with Him, you will gain power over your flesh and will grow spiritually strong. The things that tempted you before will pale in comparison to the joy of walking in obedience and enjoying sweet fellowship with Christ.

In the video *No More Sheets,* Juanita Bynum shares her experience of falling back into sexual temptation. Juanita explains the importance of "going as deep in the things of God as you were in the things of the world," not just for a season, but for a lifetime. She's had to tell some friends, "I can't do what you do… I can't go where you go… I want to be free [from sexual immorality], and I want to stay free!"

Perhaps some people might think you are legalistic for not going to an R-rated movie. Maybe your friend gets bent out of shape that you've stopped recording her soap opera for her while she's at work. Your girlfriends may think you are being a stick-in-the-mud for not going out to the singles places with them anymore. Maybe your carpool companions think you've gone too spiritual on them because you only listen to Christian music in the car.

But you know what will be evident in your life? You are a woman of conviction, and you live by those convictions. Others will see that your actions back up your words and that you give careful thought to the kind of woman you want to be. And if they ever come to realize that their lifestyles are not bringing them the fulfillment they long for, guess who they will likely run to for wise counsel? You guessed it: the woman who they know can teach them how to take every thought captive and live the overcoming life!

He will keep in perfect peace all those who trust in him, whose thoughts turn often to the Lord!

—Isaiah 26:3 (TLB)

guarding your heart

Above all else, guard your heart, for it is the wellspring of life.

PROVERBS 4:23

I once made the mistake of running a pair of my son's pants through the washer and dryer with several other articles of clothing. The problem? Rather than zips or snaps or buttons, the fly of these pants closed with a Velcro strip. Because I failed to protect the rest of my laundry by closing the Velcro flap, I ruined a silk blouse, a pair of pantyhose, and several other articles of clothing while peeling them from the Velcro's fierce grip.

Our hearts can be just like that Velcro strip. If we leave them unprotected, we make it easy for our hearts to latch on to everyone we are attracted to. Because of this, it is not enough for women to guard just our minds and bodies against sexual temptation. We also need to guard our hearts against inappropriate or forbidden relationships.

While the need to love and to feel loved is a universal cry of the heart, the problem lies in where we look for this love. If we are not getting the love we need or want from a man—whether or not we have a husband—we may go searching for it. Some look in bars and others in business offices. Some look on college campuses and some look in churches. Some women look to male friends while others look to fantasy. When love eludes them, some women seek to medicate the pain of loneliness or rejection. Some take solace in food; others in sexual relationships with any willing partner. Some turn to soap operas; others to shopping; and still others to self-gratification.

If you have tried any of these avenues for long, you have likely come to a dead end. Your pursuit has left you longing for something greater, something deeper, something more. If this has been your story, I have good news for you. God has a better way. You can seek loving, healthy relationships and guard your heart at the same time. You can find contentment with your husband and protect your heart from emotional affairs. In this chapter, we will discover:

- what God says about the heart and why you need to guard it.
- how to identify when you are about to fall into inappropriate relationships and what to do about it.
- where to discover the love that your heart yearns for.

GETTING TO THE HEART OF THE MATTER

God told us to guard our hearts above all else—above our lives, our faith, our marriage, our pocketbook, our dreams, or whatever else we hold dear. In Proverbs He tells us: "Above all else, guard your heart, for it is the wellspring of life." (4:23). Why is it so important to God that we guard our hearts?

I believe the answer is in the word *wellspring,* which can also be interpreted as "source." The heart is the source of life. When God created us, He made our hearts central to our being—physically, spiritually, and emotionally.

Physically, the heart is at the center of your circulatory system. It pumps oxygenated blood throughout your body. If there is trouble inside your heart, your entire body is in danger of losing its life-giving flow of blood. Spiritually, your heart is the place where the Holy Spirit dwells when you invite Him into your life (Ephesians 3:16-17). You receive salvation not just through head knowledge of God, but through belief in your heart that Jesus Christ is Lord (Romans 10:9-10). Emotionally, your heart leaps for joy when you find delight in something or someone. It also aches when you experience disappointment with or loss of something or someone special.

The heart is literally and figuratively the core of all you are and all you experience in life, so when God says to guard it above all else, He is saying, "Protect the source of your life—the physical, spiritual, and emotional source of your well-being." Just as a lake will not be pure if its source is not pure, neither will our thoughts, words, and actions be pure if our hearts are not pure. Purity begins in our hearts. I like how *The Message* puts it:

You know the next commandment pretty well, too: "Don't go to bed with another's spouse." But don't think you've preserved your virtue simply by staying out of bed. Your *heart* can be corrupted by lust even quicker than your *body*. Those leering looks [or thoughts] you think nobody notices—they are also corrupt. (Matthew 5:27-28, MSG, emphasis added).

Obviously, your heart needs to be a primary concern if you hope to be a woman of sexual and emotional integrity. It's one thing to determine how far is too far *physically* in a premarital or extramarital relationship, but it's another to answer how far is too far *emotionally*. What are the emotional boundaries? To help women better understand where the emotional boundaries are when it comes to relationships with the opposite sex, I developed the following models—one for single women and the other for married women. (See Figure 6.1 on the next page.)

IDENTIFYING GREEN, YELLOW, AND RED LEVELS OF EMOTIONAL CONNECTION

These models will help you identify five stages of emotional connection: (1) attention, (2) attraction, (3) affection, (4) arousal and attachment, and (5) affairs and addiction. Once you learn how to identify these stages, you can know with confidence where it's okay to let your heart go (represented by the green-light level), when to proceed only with great caution (the yellow-light level), and when you must stop and run in the opposite direction (the red-light level).

While God intends for us to enjoy our emotional connections, He did not intend for us to cross the line into a stage that would undermine our sexual and emotional integrity. Let's look more closely at each of these levels.

GREEN-LIGHT LEVEL OF EMOTIONAL CONNECTION

Attention

We've all had one of those moments when some guy catches our eye for whatever reason. Perhaps you recognize that there is a handsome man in the car next to yours at an intersection, or maybe you noticed one walking with long, steady strides down the street. Perhaps you have even experienced a certain amount of guilt for taking notice of these men, especially if you are married.

Should you be concerned if you notice an attractive man? Absolutely not. Have you gone against Scripture or broken any vows? No. Are you failing to guard your heart just because you notice that someone is eye-appealing? No. You can rest

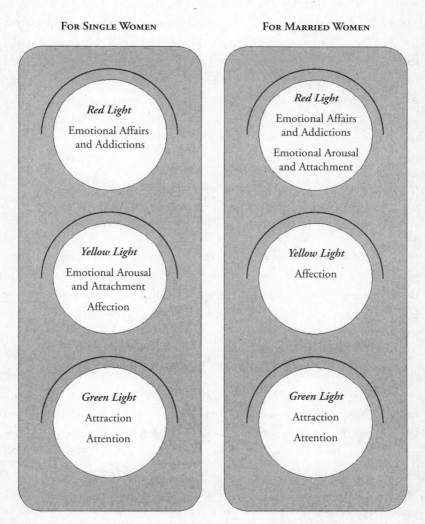

FOR SINGLE WOMEN	FOR MARRIED WOMEN
Red Light Emotional Affairs and Addictions	*Red Light* Emotional Affairs and Addictions Emotional Arousal and Attachment
Yellow Light Emotional Arousal and Attachment Affection	*Yellow Light* Affection
Green Light Attraction Attention	*Green Light* Attraction Attention

Figure 6.1: Identifying Green, Yellow, and Red Levels of Emotional Connection

easy in the fact that your eyes function very well, and you can simply thank God that He makes such fine art.

Attention is based on what we see, whereas attraction is based on what we hear. That's why I don't believe in love at first sight. It's simply *attention* at first sight. Maybe you've had the experience of noticing an incredibly handsome man, only to hear him open his mouth and yell at his kids, brag about his success, or complain about someone or something in a derogatory way. Did you find yourself attracted? No. Regardless of how gorgeous he was, you probably found yourself repulsed. He got your attention, but you felt no attraction. On the other hand, a woman can meet a very ordinary man (physically speaking) and perhaps pay little attention to him, yet she may find him very appealing upon talking with him. This is because women are stimulated more by what we hear than by what we see.

Attraction

In this stage you become familiar enough with the person to know you are drawn to him, but you are not yet familiar enough to act affectionately toward that person.

Both attention and attraction are not limited to men but can include a wide variety of things: the kind of clothes we like, the style of house we prefer, and the types of food we crave. Whether or not we feel attraction for something will determine whether we like or dislike it. It's how we know we prefer the beach instead of the mountains. It's why we have a soft spot for cuddly kittens instead of rowdy puppies. Attraction determines our inclination toward a symphony as opposed to a ballet.

We are also drawn to certain women and children. Perhaps you prefer that your child spend time with a particular playmate. You may find yourself inviting one preferred child over to play far more often than any other of your child's friends. Maybe you even go out of your way for them to play together because you so enjoy this child's company. When you go to church or business meetings, you probably are drawn to certain individuals but not to others. The woman who became your best friend is probably someone you run to when you need a hug or have really good news to share. We go through all these motions and emotions in a relationship because we feel attracted to that person.

Society has twisted our minds into thinking that if we are drawn to someone, we must want to have sex with them. But attraction isn't necessarily sexual. I find many of my friends and coworkers attractive, but I'm not the least bit tempted to have a sexual relationship with them or even an emotional affair with them.

Why are we attracted to some people and not to others? The reasons vary from person to person and are many times based on your experiences growing up. For example, I once felt a strong attraction to a family friend. I couldn't understand why until I learned about imago therapy, which teaches that certain people simply "fit your mold" and each person's mold is different. That is why you may have heard a friend rant and rave over her new boyfriend, but then you met him and thought, *What on earth does she see in him?* He fits her mold. He doesn't fit yours.

In understanding more about my own particular mold, I realized that the family friend looked very much like my brother and acted very much like my father. Of course he is going to fit my mold. Did I panic, thinking I was going to fall into an emotional affair with him because I found him attractive? I might have many years ago, but I've lived long enough to learn that attraction is all part of being human. I simply exercised caution by continuing to monitor my motives and feelings for this person.

YELLOW-LIGHT LEVEL OF EMOTIONAL CONNECTION

Affection

When you know people well enough to discern that you are attracted to them, you might feel the urge to express your feelings by showing affection or displaying favor toward them. Signs of affection may be something tangible, such as a small gift or a kind note. You could express affection by doing something beneficial for the person, like helping with a difficult task or offering to run an errand. Affection can be expressed verbally, such as by paying someone a sincere compliment or confiding in a trusted friend. We show our affection by taking time to go for a walk or going to a movie with the object of our affection. The most common expressions of affection are a pat on the back, a gentle caress, a hug, or a kiss. (Affection can, of course, progress into more sexually intimate acts.)

Gary Chapman discusses each of these forms of affection in his book *The Five Love Languages,* where he categorizes these expressions into five "languages" that can be spoken not only to spouses but also to friends and children: gifts, acts of service, words of affirmation, quality time, and physical touch.

As a married woman, you are free to show all the affection you want to the man you are married to, but what about to someone else? When is it appropriate to express affection to another man and when is it not? How do you know the difference? Where do you draw the line?

While I can't provide cut-and-dried dos and don'ts, I can suggest ways to check your heart in the matter. Prayerfully ask yourself these questions before deciding to express affection to a man other than your husband:

- What is my motive for making this expression of affection? Is it appropriate?
- Am I trying to show genuine appreciation for this individual, or do I have a hidden agenda?
- Am I using affection to draw this person into a deeper relationship?
- Could this expression be misinterpreted in such a way that this man would be confused, tempted, or suspicious of my motives?
- Is this expression of affection one that I wouldn't mind my spouse knowing about?

If you've asked God to reveal your motives and you've honestly answered each of these questions and have a clean heart, then it's probably okay to express your affection to this person. But if your motives are questionable, then don't show this person your affection. Simply treat him in a normal, friendly way and show him no preferential treatment. If you find yourself unable to limit your interactions in such a way when in this person's presence, that should be a red flag. Seek an accountability friendship to guard your heart against compromise and try to steer as clear from this person as possible until you feel more in control of your emotions.

If you are single, discerning where to draw the line can be even more confusing. If you are interested in a potentially fulfilling relationship with someone, you want to appear open without appearing desperate. If you are not interested in a romantic relationship with this person, you want to avoid sending signals that you are. And whether you are interested in a serious relationship or not, you want to avoid expressing affection in any sort of sexually provocative way. So, here are some questions a single woman should ask before expressing affection to a man:

- Is this person unattached? Does this person have a "significant other" in his life who would be concerned with how I express affection toward him?
- Is my expression of affection in line with the current level of my relationship with this person?
- Do I sense that this man has personal feelings toward me that I do not reciprocate? If so, would signs of affection give him the impression that I am interested in more than a friendship when, in fact, I am not?
- Could this expression of affection be interpreted as seductive, or does it truly reflect godly character?

If you have a clear conscience after prayerfully and honestly asking yourself these questions, then feel free to express your affection to this person in appropriate ways. But be wise if you sense your heart approaching this next level of emotional connection.

Emotional Arousal and Attachment

God has given the previous three stages (*attention, attraction,* and *affection*) for both single and married women to enjoy in a wide variety of appropriate relationships, but we must be keenly discerning about this stage. While physical arousal is easy to detect, emotional arousal can be trickier to recognize and even more difficult to control. Emotional arousal occurs when we are stirred romantically by someone, and it usually precedes most sexual activity because our heart determines the direction of our mind and body.

If you are single and hoping to develop a serious relationship with an interested, available man, emotional arousal and attachment is a natural, appropriate part of the courtship process. As you progress toward the altar, you will more than likely become deliriously excited at the thought of becoming this man's bride. There is no sin in being emotionally aroused by the man you hope to commit your life to.

But if you are married, feelings of emotional arousal and attachment toward another man are sure signs that you had better stop before you crash.

RED-LIGHT LEVEL OF EMOTIONAL CONNECTION

The only man that a married woman should feel emotionally aroused by or attached to is her husband. If you are married and you allow yourself to be emotionally aroused by and attached to another man, you are setting yourself up for compromise and even sexual sin.

How can you tell the difference between attraction or affection and emotional arousal and attachment toward a man? Here are some questions to ask yourself in order to evaluate whether or not as a married woman you are on dangerous ground:

- Do you think of this man often (several times each day) even though he is not around?
- Do you select your daily attire based on whether you will see this person?
- Do you go out of your way to run into him, hoping he'll notice you?
- Do you look for excuses to call him so you can hear his voice?
- Do you find reasons to e-mail him, eagerly anticipating his response?
- Do you wonder if he feels any attraction toward you?
- Do you want to talk or spend time alone with this person, out of earshot or eyesight of anyone else?

If the answer to any of these questions is yes, you need to stop and run in the opposite direction from this relationship until your emotions are more stable. If your feelings for this man have not been communicated to him and there is no intimacy in your relationship, you may still be able to avoid further damage by refraining from these behaviors and thought patterns. However, once feelings are communicated to this person and similar feelings are reciprocated, you've just crossed the line into an emotional affair.

If you are single and emotionally involved with a married man, or if you are married and emotionally involved with a man other than your husband, I recommend you do three things:

First, *ask God for forgiveness.* An emotional affair may not be as big a deal as a physical affair in the world's eyes, but all sin is equal in God's eyes. As you are praying for forgiveness, also ask God to reveal whether you should confess your sin to your spouse. As terrifying as this thought may be, don't let fear convince you that keeping it secret is the best thing for your marriage. (Chapter 10 will explain the benefits of confessing to your husband and hopefully give you the courage to do so.)

Next, *pray for God's divine protection,* not just over your body, but over your heart, mind, and mouth as well. Continue to pray anytime you are feeling weak or vulnerable, but make sure this person doesn't become the focus of your prayers. Instead, focus on your relationship with God, seeking to grow personally and spiritually. Pray for your other relationships with family and friends. Focus on your present blessings, and this potential burden won't look so large.

Third, *avoid any unnecessary contact with this person.* In the same way that you might have gone out of your way to cross this person's path, now go out of your way to stay out of his path. Take the long way to the restroom if the direct way passes by his office. Drive a different route so you don't pass by his house. Check your caller ID and let your answering machine screen your messages. If you are married, chances are he won't leave a message. Avoid talking privately or being alone with this person at all costs. If you have photographs displayed of this person, put them away or destroy them if they don't mean anything to anyone else. Remember, actions speak louder than words. When you refuse to remain in the presence of temptation, it loses its hold on you.

Finally, *seek a trusted friend or counselor* to hold you accountable through this season of temptation. You may choose to confide in your husband. I always run to Greg when I'm facing sexual or emotional temptation because he has a vested interest in keeping me lifted up in prayer. I also have a few female accountability relationships. If the thought of getting this honest with another woman makes you a little nervous, go back to chapter 3 and read about the last myth one more time. If you don't have a husband or a friend that you can lean on during this time of trial, it would be wise to seek professional counsel. Don't assume that your problem isn't big enough to warrant taking the time to do so. Talk about it before it gets any bigger. If you know you are going to have to answer to someone else—whether it is your husband, a friend, or a counselor—about your thoughts, words, and actions, you'll try harder to limit them to things you wouldn't be embarrassed to admit. Getting real and honest with yourself and with someone who can keep you from falling into the pit of compromise is the best lifeline available.

My experience has been that if you starve your desire to be emotionally intimate with a man, it eventually dies. The more you control your appetite for forbidden fruit, the more dignity and satisfaction you will feel about yourself and your ability to be a woman of sexual and emotional integrity.

If we don't heed the red light of a forbidden emotional attachment, we may progress toward this destructive stage of emotional connection:

Emotional Affairs and Addictions

Rather than running to the Ultimate Healer for relief from our emotional wounds, women often make idols of relationships—worshiping a man instead of God. We begin submitting to a man's and our own unholy desires rather than submitting to God's desires for our holiness and purity, thus becoming a slave to our passions.

When we peel back the layers of this issue, we can see the core problem: *doubt that God can truly satisfy our innermost needs.* So we look to a man who is not our husband and eventually discover that he doesn't "fix" us either. If we continue this pattern of looking for love in all the wrong places, we may find that our *affairs* have progressed into full-blown *addictions.*

I hope you never experience this stage—and I hope that reading this book is convicting you of your need to create a battle plan to avoid any red-light levels of emotional connection altogether. However, if you've already run the red light, please know there is hope for you. I've known many women who have journeyed to this depth of desperation, hoping to find something to fill the void in their hearts, only to discover that the pit was far deeper, darker, and more lonely than they could have imagined. I'm one of those women, but after many years of focusing my attentions and affections on my first love (Jesus Christ) and my second love (my husband), my life is a testimony to God's changing grace. In His lavish love, God's arm of mercy reaches further than we could ever fall.

Because full-blown addictions are beyond the scope of this particular book, I recommend that you see a professional counselor to discover the pain that has driven you to this point and how to heal the wounds caused by your addictive lifestyle. My earlier book, *Words of Wisdom for Women at the Well,* addresses love addictions, particularly in women, and is available at www.everywomansbattle.com or by calling 1-800-NEW-LIFE. I also recommend Stephen Arterburn's book

Addicted to Love, which addresses sex, love, romance, and relationship addictions. Here's some of what Steve has to say about this issue:

> Inevitably, romance addiction, like any other addiction, begins to interfere with the addict's life. What once brought relief soon brings pain, demanding more relief, causing more pain…and so on. What was once a technique for control takes control and throws life out of balance. The addict cannot work or play without the obsession rearing its head…. Everything else in life takes second place to feeding the addictive craving for romantic intoxication.
>
> Ironically, in almost every case the true object of the obsession is not another person, whether real or imagined, but the addict [herself]. The addict is totally focused on her own broken soul, filled with the hurts caused by all those who have abandoned her in the past. Only one thing matters: feel better now. Only one thing is sought: immediate relief from pain.
>
> Little attention or concern is wasted on anyone else. It is almost impossible for romance addicts, in the throes of their obsessive thinking and behavior, to see beyond the shell of their own self-absorption to the pain they are causing others. All they know is that they hurt, and that they must have what they need to salve their wound. If in the process they wound another, that is unfortunate. But it cannot be helped. Getting the romantic "fix" is all that matters.[1]

Again, if you feel that desperation for sex, love, romance, or relationships is something that controls your life, seek further help. You don't have to suffer in silence.

THE REWARDS OF WISDOM

As you have read through these stages and levels of emotional connection, you may have wondered if women always progress through these stages in the same order. Of course the answer is no. Any stage can be skipped over altogether. For example, a woman can engage in a private emotional affair with a man in her own mind yet never express one ounce of affection toward him. Stages can also be approached in varying order. For example, a woman may marry (attach herself to) a man for reasons other than attraction but find over time that she finds him very attractive. These exceptions are not intended to confuse you, but rather to illustrate that, while emotional connection is progressive, it doesn't always progress in the same order. Therefore, to fully guard your heart you can't assume that just because you haven't entered one stage you aren't in danger of engaging in another, more dangerous stage. Always, always check your heart for any impure motives—no matter the stage of emotional connection.

As you use caution and strive to refrain from red-light stages of emotional connection, you will regain the self-control, dignity, and self-respect you may have lost if you have compromised your sexual integrity. You can also expect a renewed sense of connection and intimacy with your husband and purity in your friendships or work relationships with other men. But best of all, when God looks on your pure heart and sees you are guarding it against unhealthy relationships, He will reward you with an even greater revelation of Himself. He says,

> I the LORD search the heart
>   and examine the mind,
> to reward a [woman] according to [her] conduct,
>   according to what [her] deeds deserve. (Jeremiah 17:10)

> Blessed are the pure in heart,
>   for they will see God. (Matthew 5:8)

Do you want a greater revelation of who God is? Do you want to experience the rewards of godly living? Do you want to experience a deeper level of satisfaction than any man can offer? Then read on as we discover the secret.

FINDING THE LOVE YOU WANT

While avoiding unhealthy emotional connections and relationships is important, it's not enough to guarantee success in keeping our hearts guarded against compromise. The secret to ultimate emotional satisfaction is to pursue a mad, passionate love relationship with the One who made our hearts, the One who purifies our hearts, and the One who strengthens our hearts against worldly temptations. The secret is to focus your heart on your First Love.

Do you remember the first time you felt you were in love? How he dominated your thoughts morning, noon, and night? How you could be available at a moment's notice if you knew he was coming by? Remember how you would drop anything and everything when the phone rang, desperately hoping to hear his voice on the line? The potential of this relationship's going somewhere consumed your world. No matter how hard you tried, you just couldn't get him off your mind, right? (Not that any of us tried all that hard!)

God longs for you to be that consumed with Him. Not that you can stay on a mountaintop like the one just described every day of your life (all love relationships go through peaks and valleys), but He desires to be your First Love. He wants your thoughts to turn to Him throughout the good and the bad days. He wants you to watch for Him expectantly, so that you sense Him beckoning you into His presence. He aches for you to call out to Him and listen for His loving reply. Although He wants you to invest in healthy relationships with others, He wants you to be most concerned about your relationship with Him.

Maybe you are thinking, *Oh, I've been hearing that all my life! The answer to all my problems is "Jesus, Jesus, Jesus!" I know Jesus but I've never felt complete satisfaction with Him, either!* If that's the case, I can understand why you might challenge what I'm saying. But I know from experience that what I say is true, and so do many women I know. And I can't help but wonder if you have really invested yourself wholeheartedly in pursuing a satisfying relationship with God. I encourage you to honestly answer the following questions:

- Have I *really* invested much time getting to know God personally and intimately?
- Do I read the Bible searching for clues as to God's character and plan for my life?
- Have I given God as many chances as I have given other men? fantasy? Internet chat rooms?

- Have I ever made the choice to pray or to dance to worship music or to go for a walk with God instead of picking up the phone to call a guy when I'm lonely?
- Are there moments spent alone (masturbating, fantasizing, reading or looking at inappropriate materials, and so on) that I ignore God's presence in an attempt to satisfy myself?
- Do I believe that God can satisfy every single need I have?
- Am I willing to test this belief by letting go of all the things, people, and thoughts that I use to medicate my pain, fear, or loneliness, and becoming totally dependent upon God?

God longs for you to test Him and try Him on this. He wants to dwell in every part of your heart, not just rent a room there. He wants to fill your heart to overflowing.

Don't let guilt from past mistakes keep you from seeking this truly satisfying first-love relationship with Him. God does not despise you for the way you've tried to fill the void in your heart. He says, "Come now, let us reason together.... Though your sins are like scarlet, they shall be as white as snow; though they are red as crimson, they shall be like wool" (Isaiah 1:18). He is eager to cleanse your heart and teach you how to guard it from future pain and loneliness.

FALLING IN THE RIGHT DIRECTION

We do not accidentally *fall* in love or into sexual immorality. We either *dive* in that direction (either passively or aggressively), or we intentionally choose to turn the other way, refusing to cross the line between that which is fruitful and that which is forbidden. Although our emotions are very powerful, we do not have to allow them to drive our thoughts and actions into compromising situations. Instead, we can fall back on God's power to guard our hearts, driving our emotions into appropriate situations and relationships.

I encourage you to memorize the green-, yellow-, and red-light levels of emotional connection discussed in this chapter. Understanding exactly where the line is between emotional integrity and emotional compromise is one of the three keys to guarding your heart. The second key is being honest with yourself and learning to recognize any hidden motives, as this will tell you exactly where you stand in relationship to that line between integrity and compromise. The third key to guarding your heart (and the most important) is pursuing a first-love relationship with Jesus Christ (which we'll talk even more about in chapter 11). Once you experience a love so pure and so passionate, your heart will be strengthened in a way that you never imagined possible.

I pray that out of his glorious riches he may strengthen you with power through his Spirit in your inner being, so that Christ may dwell in your hearts through faith. And I pray that you, being rooted and established in love, may have power, together with all the saints, to grasp how wide and long and high and deep is the love of Christ, and to know this love that surpasses knowledge—that you may be filled to the measure of all the fullness of God.

—Ephesians 3: 16-19

locking loose lips

If anyone considers [herself] religious and yet does not keep a tight rein
on [her] tongue, [she] deceives [herself] and [her] religion is worthless.

JAMES 1:26

What is a four-letter word for a woman's favorite foreplay activity? T-A-L-K!

Think about it. What affair has ever taken place without intimate words exchanged? Women often tell me, "I've not been unfaithful to my husband. All this man and I have done is talk." But what is the nature of the words exchanged? Maybe he says things like:

- "I was hoping to see your beautiful face today."
- "My wife and kids are out of town and it sure is lonely at my house."
- "I had a wild dream about you last night. Waking up was a disappointment."
- "Does your husband appreciate what a wonderful woman you are?"

Perhaps she responds with words like:

- "I just love being around you. You always make me feel good."
- "When will I see you again? Can you call me soon?"
- "I think about you all the time. I can't get you out of my mind."
- "What would your wife say if she knew we were talking like this?"

What *would* she say? What would your husband say? "It's okay, honey. You haven't been unfaithful yet"? I don't think so. Spouses would feel very betrayed by such words. As a matter of fact, those words would probably hurt just as badly as any physical acts you could have committed, because they indicate that your heart is no longer fully invested in your marriage relationship. Consider this passage from the book of James:

> When we put bits into the mouths of horses to make them obey us, we can turn the whole animal. Or take ships as an example. Although they are so large and are driven by strong winds, they are steered by a very small rudder wherever the pilot wants to go. Likewise the tongue is a small part of the body, but it makes great boasts. Consider what a great forest is set on fire by a small spark. The tongue also is a fire, a world of evil among the parts of the body. It corrupts the whole person, sets the whole course of his life on fire. (James 3:3-6)

Did you catch that last part? The tongue "corrupts the whole person." We must stop thinking about purity and faithfulness strictly in physical terms and understand the importance of matching our words, thoughts, actions, and convictions with God's Word. When all four of these things agree with one another and align with the Word of God, we are acting with sexual integrity. But if any one area is out of alignment with God's Word, we have compromised our sexual integrity, regardless of how far we've gone physically.

LINING UP OUR LIP

If we long to be women of sexual and emotional integrity, we must understand what a mighty weapon our words are. Words are what will lead us into an affair, or words will stop an affair before it ever begins.

I used to say, "I'm too weak to resist sexual temptation," and guess what? I was. But when God began dealing with me and sanctifying my mouth, I changed my tune. I started out by asking God, "Is it possible that sexual temptation could have no hold on me?" He gave me a glimmer of hope. Then I began claiming the statement, "Sexual temptation has no hold on me." After a while, I actually began believing it wholeheartedly. Now I can honestly declare with conviction, "Sexual temptation has no hold on me!"

If we tell ourselves that we can't resist sexual or emotional temptation, we will likely fall into temptation. But if we tell ourselves that we will not give in to sexual and emotional temptation, then we will be far more likely to back up our words with corresponding actions. That is how you become a woman of integrity—a person whose lip lines up with her life and vice versa.

> For out of the overflow of the heart the mouth speaks. The good [woman]
> brings good things out of the good stored up in [her], and the evil [woman]
> brings evil things out of the evil stored up in [her]. But I tell you that
> [women] will have to give account on the day of judgment for every careless
> word they have spoken. For by your words you will be acquitted, and by
> your words you will be condemned. (Matthew 12:34-37)

In this chapter we will look at guarding our mouths as further protection against sexual compromise. First, we'll examine what kind of communication to guard against—

- flirting and complimenting
- complaining and confessing
- inappropriate counseling and praying

—and then we'll look at what we can do to ensure that we guard our mouths when communicating with the opposite sex.

FLIRTING WITH DANGER

Webster's dictionary defines the word *flirt* as "to behave amorously without serious intent." Many women have asked me, "Is it okay to flirt if I'm single?" Usually the person asking this question doesn't understand what flirting really means. While it may be okay to act amorously (as if desiring romance) toward someone you are interested in developing a mutually beneficial relationship with, flirting is a different matter. Flirting could also be called "teasing," as the person doing the flirting has no serious intent. Regardless of her marital status, should a woman stir up a man (emotionally or physically) when she has no intention of pursuing a relationship with him? Is it loving to tease someone with your attentions and affections if you have no desire to fulfill any hopes you may arouse? In my opinion, showing a sincere love and respect for others allows no room for flirting or teasing.

Still others ask me, "Isn't it okay for a married woman to flirt as long as she doesn't follow through?" In my opinion, it is never appropriate for a married woman to behave amorously with anyone other than her husband. If we go back to one of our definitions of a woman of integrity, you'll remember that she lives a life that lines up with her lip, and vice versa. If we are going to be loyal to our marriage partner, we must demonstrate our faithfulness not just in our actions, but also in our communication with other people. While the saying goes, "Actions speak louder than words," we can never discount the effect that words alone have on other people and on our own integrity.

Even if you do not have serious intent when you begin batting compliments or overly friendly exchanges with a man, the excitement of those ego strokes can pull you down the road toward sexual compromise, usually slowly, but sometimes at lightning speed. Sarah found this out the hard way:

While working as a consultant for a large Christian corporation, I enjoyed sitting with a small group of other employees at banquets and company parties. We always had a great time exchanging war stories and telling jokes, some that could be repeated in mixed company and others that could not.

One evening we were all having a particularly good time in the banquet room of a restaurant and decided to continue the party at the lounge of the hotel where the out-of-town consultants were staying. As our merry group strolled into the bar, we began ordering virgin drinks and someone broke out the pool sticks and yelled, "Who's up for a game?"

As we were choosing sides, Rick (not his real name, of course) looked directly at me, winked one of his big blue eyes, and in a Humphrey Bogart–style voice said, "It's me and you, kid!" After the delightful conversation Rick and I had enjoyed over dinner and the flattering compliments he was tossing my way, I fell for that line. I remember thinking, *Lighten up and have some fun! It's a company party! And it's just a game of pool!* I called my husband and asked if I could stay out with the gang for a while.

I don't remember if we won any of the pool games or not, but I remember most of the conversation on the sidelines and how I was eating up every word. "I was hoping you'd be my partner just so we could have time to talk more…" "It's unusual to meet a woman that is smart *and* gorgeous…" "Everyone in this place has noticed what a beautiful woman I am standing next to." I also remember how Rick would slip his hand behind my waist, prompting me each time it was my turn to shoot. (I confess I was paying little attention to the game with such a smooth conversationalist by my side all evening). His touch made my insides quiver.

As the night was winding down and everyone was heading home or to his or her hotel rooms, Rick pulled me aside and slipped his hotel key into my pocket. I wish I could say that I did the right thing with that key, but I had flirted with danger for so long that night that I got reeled in, hook, line, and sinker. The conversation had been so mesmerizing. I felt as if we could have talked all night. I honestly thought that I could enter his hotel room and keep things at a conversational level, but once he kissed me we didn't do much talking.

Telling myself "At least I didn't have sex!" eased my conscience for a short time, but it didn't take long to realize that I'd packed a heavier suitcase of guilt and shame than I could carry alone. Through months of counseling, praying, and soul-searching, I realized that an affair isn't consummated when sexual intercourse takes place but when intimate conversational intercourse takes place. I just wish I had known then what I know now. I feel as if God gave me these verses specifically to keep me from deceiving myself ever again:

> But among you there must not be even a hint of sexual immorality, or of any kind of impurity…because these are improper for God's holy people. Nor should there be obscenity, foolish talk or coarse joking, which are out of place, but rather thanksgiving…. Let no one deceive you with empty words, for because of such things

God's wrath comes on those who are disobedient. Therefore do not
be partners with them. (Ephesians 5:3-4,6-7)

A FILTER FOR OUR WORDS

While many women flirt with men intentionally, others don't realize that their
amorous comments are inappropriate. We hear this kind of language so often in the
media that flirting can be a natural or automatic response. Some women are too
naïve to recognize the impact that their words and mannerisms have on the opposite sex. Other women are well aware, but are so hungry for affirmation that they
continue to jeopardize their integrity in order to fish for compliments anyway.

Here is a list of questions similar to those in the previous chapter to help you
discern whether the words that come out of your mouth and into his ears are in his
personal best interest or in the best interest of your own ego.

- What is my motive for making this comment? Is it godly?
- What do I hope to gain by saying this? Will these words be detrimental
  to either of us or beneficial to both of us?
- Is this man married? If so, would his wife get upset with me if she knew
  I was speaking to her husband in this way?
- Am I using words to manipulate this person into a deeper relationship,
  into meeting my emotional needs, or into making me feel better?
- If I actually said what I am thinking about saying, then turned around
  to find my husband (or friend, boss, pastor, or child) standing there,
  would I have some explaining to do?
- If I sense a married man is flirting with me, am I making it more fun
  for him by responding in kind, or am I maintaining my own personal
  convictions about guarding my mouth?

While kind words and compliments can be appropriate, we must be honest
about our motives and recognize when they border on becoming manipulative or
flirtatious. Even when we learn to discern whether we are flirting or not, however,
there are other forms of communication that can also lead to sexual and emotional
compromise. Let's continue examining those types of words.

COMPLAINING ABOUT THE COMPLAINING

I won't go so far to as to say that women never have a right to complain about their husbands, but such behavior with someone of the opposite sex can backfire in a hurry. Here's an e-mail I received from Beth that illustrates my point far better than I could explain it:

> When I was married, my husband emotionally abused me just about every day. Obviously not a morning person, he would wake up in a foul mood and find something to yell at me about. I let him run out of shaving cream. I didn't have his favorite shirt ironed. I didn't cook his eggs long enough. It was something every morning. He sometimes would even tell me that unless I and the house looked a little better by the time he got home he might not come home. Usually by the time I left the house for work, I felt like I had been chewed up and spit out. I would often have to sit in my car and pull myself together before going inside.
>
> I had a coworker, Bob, who saw me sitting in my car several mornings, drying my eyes before walking into the office. One day when he asked what was wrong, I didn't hold back. I confessed everything. I told him about my husband's yelling and complaining about everything I did or didn't do around the house. I confessed my hatred of how he treated me. I confessed having little love in my heart for him.
>
> Bob confessed the same frustration with his wife, saying how she didn't appreciate him either. He said he mows the lawn, takes the kids to school, washes the car, compliments her, and frequently takes her out to restaurants, but she's never happy. I thought, *Wow! If my husband did all that for me I'd melt like butter!*
>
> Bob and I began sharing marriage horror stories regularly. He became the person I vented to whenever my husband did anything to tick me off. Bob always seemed to understand and make me feel better. I'm not sure what day exactly that I fell in love with Bob, but I'll never forget the day my husband discovered our affair.
>
> I had hopes that Bob would get a divorce once my husband left, but he

decided that he could never leave his wife for the sake of their kids. He transferred to an out-of-town office so they could get a fresh start.

In hindsight, Beth realizes that two wrongs certainly didn't make a right. While her husband had no right to treat her so poorly, she only made the situation worse by complaining to another man about her husband. Beth says she wishes the only person she had complained to was a marriage counselor. At the very least, a counselor could have helped her establish some boundaries to protect herself from her husband's abusive behavior. If Beth had taken this course of action, she and her husband may have been able to work out their problems and enjoy a healthier relationship.

And speaking of counseling leads us to another form of intimate conversation that causes women to lose their emotional foothold: counseling and praying with someone of the opposite sex.

WHEN NOT TO HELP

Six days after her car wreck, Susan still could not move her head from side to side without pain radiating down her back. With the x-rays revealing no broken bones, her doctor recommended that she see a chiropractor.

Checking the yellow pages for an office close to her, Susan made an appointment for the next day. She was terrified of submitting her achy body to one who would probably bend and twist her in contortionist positions, but she prayed that God would heal her through the chiropractor's skilled hands.

"When I arrived for my appointment, I was a bit surprised to find Dr. Keifer so handsome. He had a sophisticated touch of gray along his temples and tiny laugh lines when he flashed his brilliant smile. He looked more like a *Gentleman's Quarterly* model than a chiropractor. As I lay down on the table, Dr. Keifer began the assessment with his firm touch. Six visits was his best guess, each one-week apart.

"We got to know each other pretty well during the first few visits as we shared about our families, our careers, and our mutual interests. On the fourth visit, I noticed that Dr. Keifer was not his usual jovial self," Susan explained.

"Who popped your balloon?" she jokingly asked.

"My wife, actually. Thanks for noticing my lip dragging the ground," he responded as his sweet smile began to resurface. He looked directly into her eyes as if to say, "Help me get through this!"

Susan tried to encourage him, assuring him that all would work out in time. When Dr. Keifer asked for her prayers, Susan offered to pray with him right there. He responded, "By all means," and as Susan began praying, he placed his hand on Susan's knee.

The following visit Susan inquired as to how things were on the home front. When Dr. Keifer replied that they were not so good, Susan asked, "Is there anything I can do?"

As the doctor was manipulating her spine, he also began to manipulate her heart with stories of how his wife had been so cold the past several years. Susan soaked it all in with compassionate comments sprinkled throughout the conversation. At the conclusion of her treatment, Dr. Keifer informed her that he would not be charging her for today's session because he owed her a debt of gratitude for being such a good listener.

The pleasure is all mine, thought Susan.

At the sixth and final session, the doctor reminded Susan that her insurance would pay for one more session since the last one was a freebie. Even though her neck and back were pain-free, the ache in her heart to continue seeing him drove her to go ahead and make an appointment to see Dr. Keifer again.

Too Good for Our Own Good

Women can be far too nurturing in situations, even when red flags begin to surface. We often think, *But he needs me… I'm just trying to be a friend… How can I possibly* not *help? That would not be very Christianlike!*

While it may be okay for a single woman to play the counselor role for a single male friend, if either person is married or spoken for, the plot can thicken into a dangerous recipe for relational entanglement. Or if a single woman senses that there is a hidden agenda (a desire to develop a relationship) behind a man's appeal for counsel, she would be wise not to go there at all if it's not a relationship she would care to foster.

Don't fall into the trap of counseling a man about his problems if it means having isolated personal conversations, especially if one of you is married. That is what professional counselors, pastors, and his male friends are for. The only way to avoid falling into one of the many affairs that blossom in ministry and counseling offices is for men to counsel men and for women to counsel women regarding intimate issues.

If a man comes to you for counseling or prayer and it is either a forbidden relationship or one you wouldn't consider entertaining, feel free to do what Scott did. Once approached at church by a beautiful young woman in tears, Scott responded to her in-your-face appeal for attention with a friendly, "How can I help you?"

As she proceeded to pour out her heart about something that had just upset her a great deal, Scott intuitively interrupted with, "Why don't you wait here while I get another woman to pray with you?"

Was Scott being callous? Absolutely not. He was being very sensitive, not just to the situation causing this woman's distress, but to the potential destruction of his being her sounding board and prayer partner. He did not want to feed any false hopes she may have had for a relationship with him. Many pastors and ministry leaders refuse to counsel a woman without his wife or the woman's husband present at all times. This isn't rejection; it's wise caution.

Whenever I receive requests from men asking for counsel regarding their relationship with their wife or girlfriend, I simply respond, "I'm sorry. I have a strict policy that I only counsel women. If you would like to have your wife contact me, I'd be happy to discuss matters with her and possibly see you as a couple." Wisdom tells us that if we are truly going to help other people (and protect ourselves), we cannot afford to be "too good for our own good."

Now that we've looked at what kind of communication to guard against, let's examine how we can be women of emotional integrity in all our communications with men.

STICKING TO THE BUSINESS AT HAND

It has been said that men use conversation as a means of communicating information, but women use conversation as a means of bonding. While communicating and bonding with our spouses, children, or female friends is great, communicating and bonding with men outside our marriage or with men we wouldn't choose to date is dangerous and often destructive. And yes, the more we communicate with a person, the more we bond, so we would do well to take a lesson from the men in this area and learn to stick to business a little better. We can learn to communicate with men in friendly but to-the-point ways that will not jeopardize our emotional integrity.

Whether the relationship is a forbidden one or one you simply would not want to cultivate, here are some specific guidelines to help keep your communication with other men from taking twists and turns that may ultimately lead you down the path of compromise.

Voice-to-Voice Communication

Realizing that any flame can be fanned into a raging fire by private phone conversations, try establishing these boundaries for your time on the telephone:

- If you struggle with going off on inappropriate tangents anytime you have a male listening ear, make your phone calls when other people are within earshot. If that isn't possible, set your timer for five minutes or however long you will need to tend to the business at hand. If you complete your business yet continue the conversation on a personal level, let the buzzer be your signal to close the conversation and move on to more important things.

- If calling a man from your office is a necessity, use a speakerphone. This is particularly a wise move if you are calling someone who likes to flirt with you or has sent inappropriate signals. I know it is not as personal, but that's the idea. If he suspects that other people could possibly hear everything he is saying, he'll watch every word. And the reverse is true. Pretend that you are on speakerphone and that everything you say could be monitored as well.

- If you were previously involved in a relationship and he continues to call, screen your calls using an answering machine. You are under no obligation to return a phone call to someone you want nothing more to do with, especially if he is trying to reel you back into an inappropriate relationship. If this seems incredibly rude to you, think of it as *wise* rather than rude. If you have already told him the relationship is over and he is still calling, he's the one being rude. He obviously needs a louder hint, and actions do speak far louder than words! However, if he has a valid reason for calling and you need to return his call, implement the first guideline and return the call when someone else is in earshot, or set an alarm to limit the amount of time and energy you invest in the call. This will keep you from being tempted to let him sweet-talk you back into an unhealthy relationship.

- Finally, avoid nonemergency telephone conversations past a reasonable evening hour, whether you are single or married. Remember how your parents would not allow you to talk on the phone past 10 P.M.—or whatever time? There was a good reason for that rule. Most late-night conversations are nothing but fuel for the fire.

Face-to-Face Communication

While the next chapter will address physical boundaries (discerning if and when it is ever appropriate to be alone with a particular man), we all know that situations occasionally arise before our awareness does. We show up for a doctor's appointment and his nurse steps out of the room momentarily. The electrician shows up at the house when you are the only one at home. The well-meaning neighbor stops in to see how things are going the evening your husband is away on a business trip. When such is the case, here are a few guidelines:

- Keep the topics of conversation at the same level as you would if someone else were standing there. Just because no one is in earshot, it doesn't give you an excuse to go to personal or intimate levels of conversation. As much as women like to go deep with their conversations, it isn't always wise. Before you venture into any given topic, check your motivation to make sure you don't have a hidden agenda, such as using him as a sounding board, testing his personal resolve, or looking to get your ego stroked.
- If a man tries to engage you in a conversation that seems flirtatious or even borderline (it could easily go in an inappropriate direction), respond

minimally and then find a distraction to pull you from the conversation altogether. This will send the message plainly but politely that you are not interested in playing his game.

- If a male workman shows up without a partner and you are home alone, phone a friend and ask if she can come over for a few minutes to enjoy a cup of tea—now! I have a friend in the neighborhood who shares this boundary with me, and when one of us calls the other with a spontaneous tea invitation, it's like speaking in code: *Drop everything. Come now. Tea kettle's brewing. See you in a minute.* If a friend is not available, avoid more conversation than is absolutely necessary while this man is in your home.

Computer-to-Computer Communication

With the introduction of e-mails and chat rooms, women have found cyberspace to be an extremely slippery place. Have you ever noticed that men send one or two-sentence e-mails, or sometimes even just one or two words? Women, on the other hand, send several lengthy paragraphs, the cutest poem that a friend forwarded recently, and a photo attachment of the family pet while on their latest summer vacation. While that's fine for grandma and girlfriends, let's lay down some guidelines for conversing in cyberspace with men who might tempt us toward forbidden or unhealthy relationships:

- If you must contact a man for business reasons, then stick to business. Avoid too much personal chitchat that might give the appearance that you are interested in more than just a business relationship.
- If a man that you have a previous history with or are extremely attracted to sends you an e-mail that requires a response, be very careful not to say anything that may be interpreted as being an open door or an innuendo. If this relationship causes more temptation than you can handle, you might even consider copying a third person such as your husband, secretary, or a friend for an added measure of accountability.
- Avoid private, personal e-mail accounts that no one knows about or has access to. We have a personal e-mail account and a ministry e-mail account. My husband and assistant have free access to either of these accounts anytime, providing built-in accountability.

- If a man invades your space using Instant Messenger and you sense that his intentions are less than honorable, you are under no obligation to respond at all. That's what the Do Not Accept button is for. But if you choose to respond, keep your responses brief and to the point, taking care not to veer off into a conversation that you wouldn't want someone else to be aware of.

EMOTIONAL INTIMACY WITH AN INTIMATE GOD

In our quest for relational intimacy, remember there is Someone we can whisper our heart's desires to and get our boosts from who isn't going to jeopardize our integrity but will strengthen it.

If you are thinking, *No way will talking to God ever excite me like talking to a man,* then you haven't allowed yourself to be courted by our Creator. The same God whose words possessed the power to form the entire universe longs to whisper into your hungry heart words that have the power to thrill you, heal you, and draw you into a deeper love relationship than you ever imagined possible. A guy may say that you look fine, but God's Word says, "The king is enthralled by your beauty" (Psalm 45:11). A man may tell you, "Of course I love you," but God says, "I have loved you with an everlasting love; I have drawn you with loving-kindness" (Jeremiah 31:3). Even your husband may tell you, "I'm committed to you until death," but God says, "Never will I leave you; never will I forsake you" (Hebrews 13:5).

Make time to retreat to a quiet place with the Lover of your soul. Speak whatever is on your heart, and then *listen* as God speaks straight from His heart directly to yours.

May the words of my mouth and the meditation of my heart be pleasing in your sight, O LORD, my Rock and my Redeemer.

—Psalm 19:14

building better boundaries

> Do you not know that your body is a temple of the Holy Spirit, who is
> in you, whom you have received from God? You are not your own; you
> were bought at a price. Therefore honor God with your body.
>
> 1 CORINTHIANS 6:19-20

To help us guard against temptation, Paul encourages Christians to put on the "full armor of God"—the belt of truth, the breastplate of righteousness, shoes of peace, the shield of faith, the helmet of salvation, and the sword of the Spirit (see Ephesians 6:13-17). We are so fortunate that the Holy Spirit gives us complete access to all of these things since truth, righteousness, peace, and faith are key ingredients to maintaining sexual and emotional integrity.

However, as we put on this full armor of God, women often fail to check for weak links that leave us open and vulnerable to temptation. Three of the most common weak links are:

- compromising clothing
- compromising company
- compromising actions

We'll look at each of these weak links, and as we do, try to discern if your armor may be leaving you vulnerable to temptation or jeopardizing your integrity.

WEAK LINK 1: COMPROMISING CLOTHING

You have probably heard gourmet chefs on the cooking channel say that when it comes to food, presentation is everything. Presentation *is* everything, not just with food, but also with your body. One of the concepts that I impress upon women is that *we teach people how to treat us.* We either teach them to treat us with respect or we teach them to treat us with disrespect. How? By our modest dress or our immodest attire.

After hearing me speak on the radio about the importance of modesty, Christi (in her early twenties) wrote me the following letter.

When I first began working as a Christian summer camp counselor, I decided that I would refuse to hook up with a guy at camp so that I could focus wholeheartedly on the girls in my cabin. I wanted so much for them to like me and to think I was cool, so I dressed in the latest young fashions— snug-fitting, hip-hugging jeans, short shorts, and spaghetti-strap tank tops, or tops that were short and clingy but long enough that standing still I couldn't be accused of dressing inappropriately. I also taught the girls how to do several of the latest dance moves each night in the cabin, something we all looked forward to and had a lot of fun with.

Many of the girls at camp hung around me all week instead of the other counselors. They told me how they would rather learn new dances in our cabin at night than participate in the Bible studies with their other counselors. I enjoyed thinking that I could have a big influence on these girls' lives because I had their attention and admiration.

But I also had the attention and admiration of some of the male camp counselors, which really made it hard not to get involved in a romantic relationship. I decided that I could just play it cool and clown around with these guys. They chased me around with water guns, gave me piggyback rides to the cafeteria, slipped ice down the back of my shirt and fun stuff like that.

I kept asking them to please leave me alone so I could concentrate on my girls, but they rarely respected my requests, no matter how sincere I was.

I complained to Kathy (one of the other counselors) how the guys were distracting me from what I came to do. She put her hand on mine and sweetly said, "Christi, your actions speak louder than your words. Even though you don't intend to dress to catch guys, the guys can't avoid noticing you, dressing the way you do. If you dress like a cute little plaything and present yourself as a toy, then boys will be boys and try to play with that toy!"

The magnitude of what I had done hit home the last day of camp. I noticed all of my girls rolling their shorts up to make them as short as the ones I had been wearing. They were coming up behind boys in the cafeteria and messing with them to get attention. When I noticed a group of my girls dancing in front of a bunch of boys, my first thought was, *They are a little young to be dancing like that!* But then I realized that they were only doing the dance moves that I had taught them. I had just failed to see how provocative they were. All of my best-laid plans to have a positive influence on the girls at camp had been brought to ruin by my immodest dressing and dancing.

The following year at camp, I took shorts that weren't so short and shirts long enough to be tucked in. Late at night, I taught the girls some liturgical dances to Christian music, and we even performed one in the camp talent show. The boys didn't mess with me much, so I was really able to pour a lot into the girls. I left camp that year feeling so much better about myself than the year before.

Christi's is just one of many stories I hear from women who recognize that the way they present themselves sends a nonverbal, but clear, message to men about how they want to be treated. Here are a few samples from others:

Meg, age 43:

When I was younger I used to get catcalls when I walked through the mall or through a parking lot. Now I never get any disrespect like that. When I first noticed this, I thought I must not be as attractive now that I am getting older. But I have since realized that I don't get the inappropriate attention simply because I started dressing more modestly and presenting myself like a woman on a mission from God rather than a woman on a mission to land a man.

Penny, age 32:

I used to walk around the house without much on because I was comfortable that way. I felt it was my right in the privacy of my own home. I never really thought about it until my six-year-old son brought a friend home after school one day. Bradley stopped his playmate at the door and I overheard him say, "Hold on and let me make sure my mom has some clothes on! Sometimes she doesn't." I've made it a point since then to wear something more than just underwear around the house. I don't want my children to have to explain their mother's lack of modesty!

Elizabeth, age 38:

At work my ideas would be discounted and I was passed over time after time for a promotion. It made me furious and frustrated. Then I got a revelation that if I dressed less "seductive-professional" and more "modest-professional," they might actually think I'm more than just a pretty face to decorate the office. It took awhile to gradually replace my wardrobe, but the more conservatively I dress, the more respect and appreciation I seem to get, not just from the men, but from the women as well as the clients and vendors who come into our office. I don't get propositioned when traveling nearly as much anymore either, which is good. I'd rather have the respect than the attention.

While the Bible doesn't specifically state how long a skirt should be or what sections of skin should always be covered, we can always go back to Jesus' commandment as a guideline for how we are to dress: Love your neighbor as yourself.

Picture this scenario: You know that your neighbor is dieting to lose ten pounds before her wedding. You also know that, if she does not lose the weight, her dress will be too tight and she will feel uncomfortable on her big day. But you are a gourmet dessert chef and you crave the affirmation that you are a good cook, so you insist that your neighbor eat the pound cake and fudge and coconut cream pie samples that you bring over to her house every day. Are you acting lovingly or selfishly toward your neighbor?

Now consider this: You know that men are visually stimulated at the sight of a woman's body, especially a scantily clad body. You are also aware that godly men are trying desperately to honor their wives by not allowing their eyes to stray. In light of this, if you insist on wearing clothes that reveal your sleek curves and tanned skin, are you acting lovingly or selfishly? This is a good thing to ask yourself each morning as you are getting dressed for the day. Rather than asking, "What man will I come across today and will this catch his eye?" try asking, "Would wearing this outfit be a loving expression, not causing my brothers to stumble and fall?"

Paul writes in his letter to Timothy:

> I also want women to dress modestly, with decency and propriety, not with
> braided hair or gold or pearls or expensive clothes, but with good deeds,
> appropriate for women who profess to worship God. (1 Timothy 2:9-10)

Of course, the real issue Paul was addressing wasn't braided hair or jewelry or costly clothes but rather immodesty in outward adornments. God wants us to be more concerned with our hearts than with our appearance. The story of the wife of noble character (also known as the Proverbs 31 woman) echoes the same principle but also promises that God will honor such integrity:

> Charm is deceptive, and beauty is fleeting;
>   but a woman who fears the LORD is to be praised.
> Give her the reward she has earned,
>   and let her works bring her praise at the city gate.
>   (Proverbs 31:30-31)

Remember, your figure will eventually fall south. Your skin will someday shrivel, no matter how good your moisturizer is. Your body will most assuredly return to dust. But the godly legacy of integrity and modesty that you leave behind to your children, grandchildren, and the women you influence will last far beyond the grave.

WEAK LINK 2: COMPROMISING COMPANY

As intent as we are at becoming women of sexual and emotional integrity, the company we keep can undermine our sincere efforts. While we must take responsibility for our own actions, we must also ensure that others take responsibility for their actions as well. When responsibility is refused or not taken seriously, the friend quickly becomes a foe. That's what happened to Pat.

In her midforties, Pat never expected to find herself single again. When her husband left her for another woman, she swore off men altogether. That lasted all of about three years. Then she began to feel that if a single, mature, committed Christian man crossed her path and expressed an interest in her, she would be open to exploring a new relationship. Pat writes:

Most of all, I was looking for companionship. I wanted a man who enjoyed being with me and made me laugh. When I met Michael, I felt as if he fit all my expectations. Since he was a committed Christian, I thought surely we would have the same values, including sexual boundaries. I assumed things would move slowly without pressure to get physical. Michael and I were very attracted to each other, and we talked about how it wouldn't be right to have sex outside of marriage, but we really didn't discuss any other boundaries besides that.

It became clear, however, that Michael's view on what other sexual activities were acceptable outside of marriage didn't line up with my own convictions. His gentle kisses gradually became much more passionate, and I sensed subtle pressure with his roaming hands and body massages. I realized it was up to me to draw the line and enforce the limits. But as I tried to do this, he would try to argue me back to his line. I really liked Michael, but I felt frustrated and resentful that he kept trying to wear me down. Wasn't he reading the same Bible I was? As clear as God's Word is about avoiding even a hint of sexual immorality, I wondered why we were even having these discussions!

I finally had to walk away from this relationship. Unfortunately, by that time I'd given him my heart, and walking away, although it was the right thing, was incredibly hard to do. He calls every once in a while to see if I'll give him another chance, but I just don't think he's good company for me to keep if he can't respect my personal boundaries.

Pat valued herself too much to be totally taken advantage of and coerced into completely abandoning her morals and values. She says, "I'll be a lot wiser next time, not just about my body, but also about my heart." Fortunately, Pat realized that Michael was taking her for granted by trying to push her further than her personal convictions would allow.

When you spend time with someone, you are giving that person a gift: *your presence.* It's true. The gift of your company is very precious and of value beyond description. Underneath your breasts lies a beating heart where the Holy Spirit makes His home. Behind your face is a brain that possesses the mind of Christ. Be wary of men who are intrigued by the wrapping but fail to see the value of what is inside the package. They may want to play with the bow...untie the ribbon...peek through the wrapping.

I'll never forget my daughter's first Christmas. At nine months old, she was enamored with the packages and bows. We had to put the Christmas tree in a playpen to keep her from unwrapping every present. With each gift given by family members, Erin would rip into the package with utter delight, toss the gift aside, and play frantically with the paper, bows, and ribbons.

Many men do the exact same thing with women. Although the gift inside (her heart and soul) is of great worth, the wrapping is what holds their interest and motivates their actions. Men who value the wrapping (her body) more than the gift inside are bad company. As women of great worth, pearls of great price, we have every right to refuse to grace them with our presence, and we must learn to exercise this right as Joseph did with Potiphar's wife:

Now Joseph was well-built and handsome, and after a while his master's wife took notice of Joseph and said, "Come to bed with me!"

But he refused. "With me in charge," he told her, "my master does not concern himself with anything in the house; everything he owns he has entrusted to my care. No one is greater in this house than I am. My master has withheld nothing from me except you, because you are his wife. How then could I do such a wicked thing and sin against God?" And though she spoke to Joseph day after day, he refused to go to bed with her or even be with her. (Genesis 39:6-10)

Can you imagine a slave being bold enough to refuse to even be in the presence of his master's wife? Obviously, Joseph knew that bad company corrupts good character. He was a man of great courage and integrity, and God eventually blessed him richly and entrusted a great deal into his care because of his integrity.

But what about you? Ask God to give you this kind of courage and integrity. Determine not to give away the gift of your presence to anyone who wants it. Remember, you are a pearl of great price, a woman to be treasured. By being careful about the company you keep, you can ensure that your temple of the Holy Spirit is well protected.

WEAK LINK 3: COMPROMISING ACTIONS

Before getting married and settling down thirty years ago, Terri frequented local country-western dance halls with friends for weekend entertainment. Friday and Saturday nights were filled with many handsome boot-scooters, a few mixed drinks, and an occasional one-night stand. "Once I got married, going out to nightclubs to dance was something that my husband and I did only on rare special occasions," Terri reminisced with a tone of regret.

Since becoming a widow two years ago at the age of fifty-three, Terri has often been invited to go out dancing with girlfriends from work. Tired of sitting around and feeling sorry for herself, she finally gave in. "The weekends are a particularly lonely time for me. I thought it would be good to get out of the house and back out onto the dance floor for some fun and exercise."

Slipping her slender figure into her starched Wrangler jeans, Terri took pride in how attractive she still was at her age. No doubt she would be asked to dance many times before the night was through.

Walking into the honky-tonk, Terri's heart pounded in sync with the base guitar, and her eyes twinkled as her gaze followed the colorful spotlights bouncing across the room. She and her friends struggled through the crowd to find an unoc-cupied table and settled onto the tall stools to order a round of drinks. Before her strawberry margarita had even arrived at the table, a tall gentleman in a dashing black cowboy hat leaned over her shoulder and shouted over the music into her ear, "Hello, ma'am. I'm Brett and I'd love to have this next dance!"

Glancing at her friends and grinning with delight, Terri took Brett's hand and shuffled out to the center of the floor where he wrapped one arm around her petite waist and cupped her hand in the palm of his own. Pressing his cheek against hers, Brett escorted her around and around with a two-step shuffle and an occasional twirl that sent her mind and her heart reeling with excitement.

Midnight came quickly and after many dances and a few drinks, Brett asked if he could see her home. "My friends from the office would never let me hear the end of it if I didn't go home the same way that I came," Terri replied. Flattered by his obvious disappointment, she scribbled her phone number on a napkin and slipped it into his shirt pocket. Reluctantly, she turned to walk out of the beams of the neon moon to return home with her girlfriends, hoping that maybe Brett would invite her out the following weekend.

Terri walked into her dark house, dreading another lonely night sleeping single in a double bed. Making her way into the kitchen to check her messages, she was startled when the phone rang. Pleasure washed over her at the sound of Brett's voice. Still under the influence her margaritas, she agreed to have him over for a little while now that her girlfriends would never know.

Sadly, Terri's compromising actions may lead her to discover what many women who are returning to the dating scene are finding out the hard way: *It is not the same scene as it was many years ago.* Up until the 1970s, researchers were only aware of two significant types of sexually transmitted diseases (STDs): syphilis and gonorrhea. Both of these diseases were easily cured with a shot of penicillin, so STDs weren't much of a deterrent from sexual activity.

Today however, researchers estimate there are twenty to twenty-five significant types of sexually transmitted diseases, only a few of which will be discussed here. A panel of experts reported the following estimates for incidence, prevalence, and cost of STDs in the United States:

- 15 million new cases of sexually transmitted disease occur each year in Americans.
- The current prevalence of STDs is over 68 million.
- The yearly direct cost of STDs is just over $8 billion.
- The STD that currently infects the most Americans is genital herpes (45 million).
- The STD with the highest yearly incidence of new infections is human papillomavirus (HPV) (5.5 million).[1]

One of the STDs that receives a lot of press is HIV, which eventually develops into AIDS and is of course deadly. While AIDS prevention efforts have historically targeted gay men and teenagers, in some areas of the country the highest rate of heterosexual transmission of AIDS occurs in people over fifty. *Yes, I said people over fifty years old.* In Palm Beach County, Florida, one of the most popular areas for retirees, the rate of HIV infection for elderly persons shot up 71 percent between 1992 and 1993.[2]

If we weren't hearing so much about HIV, we would hear a lot more about HPV. This disease has the highest annual rate of infection (again, 5.5 million people each year in the United States alone). While bacterial infections can be treated with antibiotics, there is no medical cure for viral infections such as HPV, herpes, and HIV. Symptoms of viral infections can be treated, but ultimately the virus stays with you for life. Here is what the Medical Institute for Sexual Health (MISH) has to say about HPV:

- HPV is the virus present in over 93 percent of all cervical cancers.
- More women die from cervical cancer than die from AIDS each year in the United States.
- Most Americans, including American health-care professionals, are currently unaware of HPV's dramatic prevalence. In addition to cervical cancer, HPV can lead to vaginal, vulvar, penile, anal, and oral cancer.
- Dr. Richard Klausner of the National Cancer Institute has stated, "Condoms are ineffective against HPV because the virus is prevalent not only in mucosal [wet] tissue, but also on dry skin of the surrounding abdomen and groin, and can migrate from those areas into the vagina and cervix."[3]

MISH estimates that 70 to 80 percent of the time an STD carrier will have absolutely no symptoms. Without proper medical testing, you may never know you have the disease, but you can certainly pass it on to any partner you come in contact with. Many of these diseases are your companions for life and will more than likely cause infection in anyone you have any type of sexual activity with (vaginal, oral, or anal sex or mutual masturbation).

Certain segments of society have convinced many people that if you have protected sex ("safe sex"), you won't have to fear disease. While using a condom may make sex more safe than completely unprotected sex, condoms by no means make sex *safe*. In a study to determine if condoms protect against the spread of the HIV virus, researchers estimate that condoms are effective only 69 percent of the time. That leaves a 31 percent risk factor. Dr. Susan Weller is quoted as saying, "It is a disservice to encourage the belief that condoms *will prevent* sexual transmission of HIV."[4]

The only way to truly protect yourself is to guard against sexual compromise altogether. No condom fully protects you against the physical consequences of sexually immoral behavior. Even more important, no condom protects you against the spiritual consequences of sin (broken fellowship with God). No condom will protect you from the emotional consequences of a broken heart. Therefore, don't think in terms of "safe sex," but in terms of "saving sex" until marriage or remarriage. Wise is the woman who avoids compromising behavior that can put her body at risk of disease.

If this revelation is coming after you've allowed your physical boundaries to be crossed, do yourself a favor and go to a doctor for an STD screening. Treatment may save your life and the lives of others.

A FEW MORE BOUNDARIES

If you guard your body against the weak links of compromising clothes, compromising company, and compromising actions, and integrate the boundaries for your thoughts, emotions, and words as discussed in the previous chapters, you should have a full armor of protection. But before we close our discussion on guarding our bodies, here are a few other personal boundaries to consider:

- Save your hugs for girlfriends and immediate family members. Rarely is a hug absolutely necessary with a male friend when a handshake, a pat on the back, or a smile will do. If you decide that a hug is appropriate, give a "brother hug" which is initiated standing beside a person with your arm around his shoulder for a quick side-by-side squeeze or pat on the back. If a man comes at you face to face and initiates a hug unexpectedly, simply lean your body forward so that he hugs your neck rather than your body.

- When venturing anywhere, whether it is across town, across the campus, or across the hallway, make sure you do not go out of your way to run into guys who always compliment you or make you feel good. Certain gentlemen are extremely fun to be with, and it is easy to be tempted to place ourselves in their path just to get our emotional basket filled or our ego stroked. But putting ourselves in their path also means walking down Temptation Trail. Remember, "When in route, stay on course!"

- Many men and women of integrity have decided never to be alone with a member of the opposite sex without a third person within eyesight and earshot. Billy Graham tells of how he has another man escort him from meetings into his hotel room so that he is never in a situation where he may have to converse with a woman one on one. God has obviously honored this boundary with a fruitful ministry, and I'm sure Mrs. Graham has appreciated Billy's integrity as well! If no provision is ever made to be alone with a man, an affair would be difficult to conduct, and it is just as important for Christians to avoid the *appearance* of evil as it is to avoid evil itself.

- Be selective about who you ride in a car alone with. The inside of a car is an extremely intimate place (as many of us discovered when we first began car dating!). The feeling of isolation and seclusion from the rest of the world while in an enclosed car provides the perfect environment for inappropriate thoughts or actions to blossom.

- Always keep the door open when in a man's office, and keep your door propped open if a male coworker enters your office. I know one supervisor who installed a glass door on her office so that when male employees wanted to speak privately with her there was never a question as to what was going on behind her closed door.

Remember that your body is the temple of the Holy Spirit; your heart, God's dwelling place. As a believer, you have the mind of Christ. And your words are instruments of His wisdom and encouragement to others. When you put on the full armor of God and vigilantly guard your body, heart, mind, and mouth without compromise, you are well on your way to reaping the physical, emotional, mental, and spiritual benefits of sexual integrity.

Do not be deceived: God cannot be mocked. A [woman] reaps what [she] sows. The one who sows to please [her] sinful nature, from that nature will reap destruction; the one who sows to please the Spirit, from the Spirit will reap eternal life.

—Galatians 6:7-8

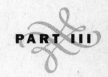

PART III

embracing victory in retreat

sweet surrender

> Do not let any part of your body become a tool of wickedness, to be
> used for sinning. Instead, give yourselves completely to God since you
> have been given new life. And use your whole body as a tool to do what
> is right for the glory of God.
>
> ROMANS 6:13 (NLT)

Mindy, a participant in one of my Well Women growth groups came into my
office near her wit's end:

> I'm not acting out sexually anymore, but I'm really struggling with other
> issues. I don't know what is going on, but I can't seem to get along with any
> of my roommates. I can't stand to be with them, but I can't stand to be
> alone, either. I hate what I see when I look in the mirror. [Mindy is a strik-
> ingly beautiful young woman]. I feel stressed, anxious, and angry most of the
> time, but I don't know why. I can't sleep at night and my heart keeps racing.
> I've been sick with one thing or another for months, but when I went to the
> doctor for a checkup, he couldn't find anything wrong. I'm having the same
> kind of suicidal thoughts I had before when I was in a mental institution.
> Can you help me?

Considering the gravity of Mindy's words, I wasn't sure I could. I'm not a
trained psychologist, so I encouraged her to talk with a professional on campus.
Then I asked if we could talk. Mindy claimed she was faithful to her quiet times,
had no dealings with any substance abuse, was eating a relatively healthy diet, and

had forgiven all of her former boyfriends as well as her parents and siblings for any wrongs she felt they had done to her. "There is no one left to forgive. I've gone through the list over and over in my head," Mindy insisted.

Now at *my* wit's end as to what could be troubling her so, I ended our session with a prayer. "God, please give us clear insight as to what is going on in Mindy's mind, heart, and body and give us discernment as to how to remedy this situation," we pleaded.

I got in my car and drove down the road to Mercy Ships International headquarters where I was late for a discipleship training class. Our speaker for the day was Pastor Mel Grams, whose lecture on forgiveness was already underway. As he shared the following information from an article in the January 1999 issue of *Prevention* magazine, I was amazed. The symptoms related to unforgiveness directly paralleled Mindy's symptoms.

According to this article, psychologists report that unforgiveness causes negative feelings about people in general, failure to recognize and enjoy potentially good relationships, and the following psychological problems:

- chronic anxiety
- serious depression
- general mistrust
- poor self-esteem
- anger and hatred
- resentment

In addition, physicians also cited the following physical consequences of unforgiveness:

- rush of hormones exhilarate heart rate
- limits or shuts down immune system
- chances of heart attack increase by 500 percent
- risk of high blood pressure and cholesterol
- enhances risk of blood clots and cancer
- a host of other chronic issues[1]

Sensing there had to be more to this scenario, I prayed again, "Lord, why does Mindy have so many of these exact symptoms even after she has forgiven everyone who has ever hurt her?" Then it clicked. She had forgiven everyone else. But had she forgiven *herself*?

I copied my notes frantically and took them to the growth group that evening to discuss them with Mindy afterward. "Do these sound like the symptoms you are suffering from?" Reading the list, she replied yes to most of them. I said, "Mindy, these are what psychologists and physicians say unforgiveness does to a person. You mentioned having forgiven everyone you could imagine, but have you forgiven yourself?"

Her big brown eyes filled with tears before she could get the words out. "No, and I don't know if I'll ever be able to," she cried.

LETTING GO OF PAST EMOTIONAL PAIN

If you want to win the battle for sexual integrity, you must let go of past emotional pain. Maybe a father who was absent, either emotionally or physically, wounded you. Maybe the distance in your relationship with your mother left you feeling desperately lonely. Perhaps your siblings or friends never treated you with dignity or respect. If you were abused in any way (physically, sexually, or verbally) as a child, maybe you have anger and pain that has yet to be reconciled.

Perhaps old lovers took advantage of your vulnerabilities, strung you along, or were unfaithful to you. Or maybe you've never understood why God allowed——— to happen (you fill in the blank). Regardless of its source, we must surrender the pain from our past in order to stand strong in the battle for sexual and emotional integrity.

It took me a long time to let go of the pain of losing my eight-year-old sister when I was only four and to forgive God for allowing her death. I had difficulty forgiving the eighteen-year-old boy who coerced me into bed when I was only fourteen. And it took me years to release the bitterness and anger I felt toward my father for being so emotionally disconnected from me. I eventually found God's grace for every person who had ever left me, let me down, or offended me in any way. But forgiving myself for the poor choices I'd made throughout my life seemed to require far more grace than I could muster. Whenever I would reflect on what

I'd done, I would think, *I can't believe how stupid I've been. I should have known better. No one could possibly love me if they knew all the things I've done.*

Little did I know that these kinds of thoughts made me more vulnerable to emotional and sexual temptations. My self-esteem was in the gutter, so I continually sought affirmation from outside sources, especially older men. I felt exactly the way Mindy did—I hated what I saw in the mirror each day—and I hoped that if men thought that I was attractive, then maybe I could believe it too. But even finding a husband didn't solve my problem. It wasn't enough to have a man who thought the world of me. Even with a wedding band on my finger, my antenna was still up to see who was noticing me. And when my radar went off and I knew that someone had me in his range, I was too often a sitting duck. I'd say to myself, *You may as well give in. You know how you are when you are tempted. What's one more time?*

One day as I was beating myself up for yet another emotional affair, my best friend interrupted me with these sobering words: "Do you know what you are saying about the blood that Jesus shed for you when you refuse to forgive yourself for your past? You are saying that His blood wasn't good enough for you. It didn't have enough power to cleanse you." She was right. Underlying all of my self-pity was the belief that what Jesus did for me couldn't possibly be enough to rid me of my stain. I needed some special miracle to set me free, and until I got that miracle, I had to beat myself up as an act of penance.

If this rings true for you as well, then guess what? The Holy Spirit is telling you the same thing He told me back then: *Jesus opened your prison door. It's up to you to walk out!* How do you do this? By forgiving every person who has ever brought you pain, including yourself. If God does not despise you for the ways you have tried to fill the void in your heart, neither should you despise yourself. Paul preached, "Righteousness from God comes through faith in Jesus Christ to all who believe. There is no difference, for all have sinned and fall short of the glory of God, and are justified freely by his grace through the redemption that came by Christ Jesus" (Romans 3:22-24).

In other words:

- Righteousness does not come from perfect living, but as a gift
  from God.

- We receive this gift not by our worthiness, but simply by faith in Jesus Christ (and in the blood He shed for the redemption of our sins).
- We are justified freely by God's grace—no strings attached.

When I am justified, it is "*just-as-if-I'd* never done those things." So why do we continue beating ourselves up? Why do we allow our misery to affect our mental and physical health? You don't have to carry all that emotional baggage. Surrender your pain and your backpack full of guilt and shame; it is only making you tired and crabby. Travel light and let the joy of the Lord be your strength! Letting go of bitterness fosters healthy changes in our attitudes, promotes healthy changes in our bodies, lowers blood pressure and heart rate, boosts self-esteem, and gives feelings of hope and peace.

Forgiveness is essential not just for emotional and physical healing, but also for true worship. Matthew 5:23-24 says, "Therefore, if you are offering your gift at the altar and there remember that your brother has something against you, leave your gift there in front of the altar. First go and be reconciled to your brother; then come and offer your gift." In other words, God desires our reconciliation with one another before we come to Him in worship. I believe that not only does He desire our reconciliation with one another, He wants us to be reconciled to ourselves as well.

When we don't forgive, we are blocked spiritually. We can't grow. In 2 Corinthians 2:10-11, Paul writes, "If you forgive anyone, I also forgive him. And what I have forgiven—if there was anything to forgive—I have forgiven in the sight of Christ for your sake, in order that Satan might not outwit us. For we are not unaware of his schemes." Here Paul warns that Satan uses unforgiveness as a tool to bring about our destruction. Forgiveness foils Satan's plots to stunt our spiritual growth.

To enter the process of forgiveness, you must take these steps:

- Acknowledge your anger and hurt. It is very real and God knows it is there.
- Realize that holding on to this pain only holds you back.
- Consciously let go of any need for revenge.
- Consider the source of your pain: Hurting people hurt other people. Put yourself in their shoes.
- Pray earnestly for those who hurt you, asking God to heal the wounds that cause them to wound others.
- Pray that your wounds do not cause you to do the same to others.[2]

I walked through each of these steps in the process of forgiving my father, my husband, every other man who hurt me and was eventually able to forgive myself as well. As a result, I finally got over the barricade that had separated me from fully experiencing the love of my Savior for so long.

Not only do we need to surrender past emotional pain so that our hearts can receive the love God wants to lavish on us, we also must surrender our pride.

RELINQUISHING PRESENT PRIDE

One of the first complete sentences my daughter learned to formulate as a toddler was, "Me do it by mine elf." I applauded Erin's desire to be self-sufficient, except when her desire to be independent outweighed her ability to manage on her own.

She often refused to hold my hand while walking because she wanted to walk by herself. Occasionally she would momentarily get lost in the shuffle of a crowd or would fall facedown on the sidewalk, crying for Mommy or Daddy to pick her up. While this may sound like irresponsible parenting, we knew that forcing her to hold our hand would teach her nothing. Allowing her to stumble and fall a little would teach her not to be too proud to ask for help when she needed it. Our heavenly Father does the same with us. He never *forces* us to take His hand but allows us to experience the need for His hand so that we will *desire* it. When we tell ourselves, *I can handle this battle on my own, I don't need help, I can manage without accountability,* we set ourselves up for a fall.

I recently heard a statement that made my heart skip a beat: "You are never more like Satan than when you are full of pride." Isn't it true? Pride got Satan expelled from heaven. Pride hinders sinners from asking Jesus to be their Savior and submitting to His Lordship. And pride keeps Christians from repenting from the things that cause them to stumble and fall, such as sexual and emotional compromise.

The consequences of pride can be truly devastating. Eve's pride got her expelled from the Garden of Eden when she was deceived into believing, *I can be as wise as God if I eat this fruit.* When Moses was leading God's people through the desert, he assumed that God needed his help when he asked the Israelites, "Must we bring you water out of this rock?" (Numbers 20:10). This failure to honor God as the only one capable of such a miracle disqualified Moses from being the leader who would actually usher the people into the Promised Land. When David peered down from his roof at Bathsheba, he must've said to himself, "I am the king, and the king gets whatever the king wants." His pride led him to commit adultery with Bathsheba and then murder her husband, Uriah, by sending this loyal commander to the battlefront to ensure that he would die. I'm sure Eve, Moses, and David would testify that sometimes pride can rear its ugly head and bite you before you even recognize it has invaded your heart. Therefore, in this battle for sexual and emotional integrity, it is important that you learn to recognize pride and repent of it before you take a fall.

Here are some illustrations of how pride can make us vulnerable to sexual and emotional temptation:

- Although she is married, Carla claims it's no big deal when her friend Danny flirts and jokes around with her. When he tosses out some sexual innuendos, she responds in kind, insisting that any woman would do the same. *Translation: The rules of right and wrong don't apply to me. I can bend the standards of righteousness because others do it as well.*

- Once active in an accountability group, Alicia has stopped attending because of the time she spends with her new boyfriend, Rob. Concerned about her sudden disappearance, Alicia's friend from the group has tried to call several times just to make sure Alicia is staying grounded in her commitment to keep God first in her life and not get sucked into another sexual relationship. Alicia finds the calls annoying, refuses to pick up the phone, and wishes everyone would just leave her and Rob alone. *Translation: I don't need anyone holding me accountable. I'm above temptation or reproach. What I do is nobody else's business.*

- Shirley's premenstrual moods have driven her husband of fifteen years further and further away. To compensate for her lack of emotional connection, her conversations with a friendly male coworker have gotten more and more intimate. *Translation: If I can't get my emotional needs met by my husband, I'll get them met elsewhere.*

Pride assumes several things:

- I deserve whatever I desire.
- My needs should be met at any cost.

- Life is all about me and my pleasure.
- The rules apply to everyone else but me.
- I'm above the consequences.

While we may never say these statements out loud, don't our actions some-times prove these attitudes to be true?

If we long to be women of sexual and emotional integrity, we must surrender our pride. James 4:6 reminds us that "God opposes the proud but gives grace to the humble." We can imagine what being opposed by God might look like (and shudder at the thought!). But what does God's "grace to the humble" look like? Titus 2:11-14 describes it vividly:

> For the grace of God that brings salvation has appeared to all men. It teaches
> us to say "No" to ungodliness and worldly passions, and to live self-
> controlled, upright and godly lives in this present age, while we wait for the
> blessed hope—the glorious appearing of our great God and Savior, Jesus
> Christ, who gave himself for us to redeem us from all wickedness and
> to purify for himself a people that are his very own, eager to do what
> is good.

Do you want to be able to say no to worldly passions? to live a self-controlled, upright, and godly life? to be purified as God's very own? to be eager to do what is good? You can't do these things "by mine elf!" as Erin used to say. But God can give you what you need when you humble yourself before Him and say, "I surrender my pride. I need help if I am to experience Your plan for my sexual and emotional fulfillment, and I'm willing to be held accountable for my actions."

Then keep your eyes open for that accountability partner. Perhaps it will be a friend or a sister, a teacher, a counselor, or a mentor. While you may be tempted to look for someone who can sympathize with you, you may have more long-term success with someone who isn't struggling herself or who has already overcome such a struggle. Hitching two weak oxen together to plow a field is not nearly as effective as hitching a weak ox with a strong one.

When you have a mentor who can show you how to thrive on a diet of humil-ity, you may discover a healing change in your appetite. Remember, we can not sin and win. If there is sexual or emotional sin in your life, you must starve it to death. You can't just "trim it down" or it will just grow right back, even larger than before. Sin must be cut out completely.

But perhaps you are wondering if you even *want* to cut some habits out altogether. Maybe you really *like* doing what you are doing or thinking what you are thinking.

One of the most honest prayers I've ever heard is, "Lord, forgive me for the sins that I enjoy!" Sin often feels good (at least initially), or else it wouldn't be tempting. But recognizing how your pet sins ultimately impact your life may inspire you to surrender them.

When we humbly submit to the Gardener's shears and allow Him to cut out pride so we can grow, our attitude will begin to move in the opposite direction:

- While pride says, "I deserve whatever I desire,"
  humility says, "My fleshly desires will not dictate my actions."
- While pride says, "My needs should be met at any cost,"
  humility says, "Meeting my needs is secondary to loving others."
- While pride says, "Life is all about me and my pleasure,"
  humility says, "Life is all about God and His pleasure."
- While pride says, "The rules apply to everyone else but me,"
  humility says, "I will submit to the rules for righteousness' sake."
- While pride says, "I'm above the consequences,"
  humility says, "I win only when I resist sin."

In addition to letting go of emotional pain and learning to exchange pride for humility, we must surrender our fears of the future if we want to protect ourselves from sexual and emotional compromise.

FEAR OF THE FUTURE

Have you ever counted how many references there are to *fear* in Scripture? Three hundred and sixty-five (one for every day of the year!). As many times as God proclaimed, "Fear not..." it is obvious that fear is a major hindrance to the Christian life.

Why is it such a hindrance? Because *fear* is the opposite of *faith*. When we focus on our fear rather than having faith in God to deliver us from evil, we are much more likely to lose the battle for sexual and emotional integrity. How can we focus on what we know God will do when we think we are doomed? Such lack of faith says to God, "Even though you've carried me this far, you are probably going to fail me now, aren't you?" Overcoming our fear and exercising our faith says to God, just as David did in Psalm 9:9-10, "The LORD is a refuge for the oppressed, a stronghold in times of trouble. Those who know your name will trust in you, for you, LORD, have never forsaken those who seek you."

I love taking youth groups to a high-ropes challenge course. There we gear up with helmets and safety pads and are connected to a guide wire in order to waltz across a twelve-foot balance beam suspended twenty-five feet in the air between two telephone poles. This exercise can bring out the lion in the most timid of creatures and the mouse in the boldest. I've seen dainty young girls saunter up the pole and tiptoe across gracefully without breaking a sweat. I've also seen two-hundred-pound linebackers turn white with fear and break out in tears midway through the course.

Before they climb the telephone poles, I always ask, "Would you have a problem walking across a wooden beam that was two inches off the ground?" When they say no, I remind them that walking across a beam twenty-five feet in the air is physically no different. The only difference is the mental challenge of overcoming the fear of heights. Success comes when we tune out the surroundings and focus on putting one foot in front of the other.

The same is true in our battle against sexual and emotional compromise. Many women are steeped in the fear of being alone, the fear of not being taken care of, the fear of not having another man on the hook in case the current one gets away. We can be so afraid of compromising tomorrow that we fail to take notice and celebrate the fact that we are standing firm today.

For example:

- Helen says, "Bill is not someone I am really interested in because he's too touchy-feely, but whenever a weekend comes around that I don't have plans, I usually accept his dinner invitation because I just can't face a whole weekend alone."

- Married eight years, Barb isn't sure she and Jim are going to make it. They argue frequently and Barb is bitterly disappointed over Jim's callous style of relating to her. "When I get really upset with him, I always know I can cry on Charlie's shoulder." (Charlie is Barb's old boyfriend who always wanted to marry her.) "I have kept all of Charlie's love letters and our old pictures together. I'm afraid to get rid of them. After all, he might someday be 'the one' if Jim and I don't work out."

- Since her husband died two years ago, Beatrice worries about her financial situation. "I don't feel that I am ready to invest in a new relationship and am not even sure I ever want to remarry," Beatrice says. However, she thinks she may have to begin dating again because she may eventually need a husband to provide for her.

I used be overwhelmed at the thought of long-term, lasting fidelity. I often thought, *Oh, there's no way I can be faithful to one man for an entire lifetime!* When a mentor asked me, "Can you be faithful for one day?" I scoffed at the ridiculousness of the request. "Of course I can. One day is no big deal! It's the rest of my life that I'm worried about."

"Life consists of one twenty-four-hour period after another. If you can be faithful for one day, you've got it made," my mentor responded. "You just do the same thing the next day and the next day."

The simplicity of her response floored me. Taking one day at a time and trusting our future to God *is* all it takes. That's why Jesus taught us to pray, "Give us today our daily bread." That is why God rained down bread from heaven each day when the Israelites were wandering in the desert without food—so that His people would learn *daily* dependence on Him. When we change our focus from the distant future to the immediate present, we gain the strength and courage to overcome the fear of what we may encounter down the road. Don't focus on whether you can be faithful to one man for a lifetime—just focus on being faithful to him (or to God if you are single) just for today. Then do the same thing tomorrow, and the next day, and the next.

WAVING THE WHITE FLAG

Waving a white flag in the midst of battle is a symbol of surrender. A white flag symbolizes that the troops are no longer posting their own colors, but a neutral color as a sign of defeat. However, the white flag you will be waving as you surrender your past pain, present pride, and future fear is *not* a symbol of defeat. It is a symbol of victory, for it represents purity. You will be washed clean of all compromise as you allow God to transform you—heart and mind—into a woman who forgives her debtors, walks in humility, and faces the future with confidence in her Creator and Sustainer.

White is your color, girlfriend! Post it proudly and enjoy the peacefulness and fulfillment of sweet surrender to the Savior.

But the wisdom that comes from heaven is first of all pure; then peace-loving, considerate, submissive, full of mercy and good fruit, impartial and sincere. Peacemakers who sow in peace raise a harvest of righteousness.

—James 3:17-18

rebuilding bridges

For this reason a man will leave his father and mother and be united
to his wife, and they will become one flesh. The man and his wife were
both naked, and they felt no shame.

GENESIS 2:24-25

The banking industry invests a considerable amount of time training their employees to recognize counterfeit bills. Rather than introducing a variety of counterfeits and teaching employees how to recognize those, they have employees spend a great amount of time handling nothing but genuine currency. The logic is that if they know the real thing by heart, they'll never accept an imitation.

The same principle applies to intimacy in marriage. Once you understand what a priceless gift your sexuality is and how it can bond you and your husband in a way that you'll never experience outside of marriage, you'll be far less likely to settle for anything less than God's plan for sexual and emotional fulfillment.

However, both men and women have handled counterfeit intimacy for so long that they've lowered their standards and settled for far less than the real thing. Men look for satisfaction through sex, but physical intimacy alone doesn't bring ultimate fulfillment. Many women can attest to the fact that just because a man is fantastic in bed doesn't mean he fulfills her emotionally. Even great sex in marriage is not the same as genuine intimacy.

On the other hand, we look for satisfaction through emotional connection, but this will not fulfill us unless it's celebrated through physical intimacy with our spouse. A sexless marriage resembles a friendship more than a marriage. Because sexual tension typically builds much faster for men than for women, we'll more than likely have this friendship with a very sexually frustrated husband. Even the deepest emotional connection is no substitute for genuine intimacy.

Genuine sexual intimacy involves all components of our sexuality—the physical, mental, emotional, and spiritual. When these four are combined, the result is an elixir that stirs the soul, heals the heart, boggles the mind, and genuinely satisfies.

How unfortunate are those who have never tasted the sweetness of sexual intimacy as God intended it to be because they have accepted one or two parts as a counterfeit for the whole. Fulfillment never comes to those who insist, "He doesn't meet my emotional needs, so why should I meet his physical needs?" or "She doesn't even try to understand my physical desires, why should I bother trying to understand her emotional desires?"

When you first picked up this book subtitled *Discovering God's Plan for Sexual and Emotional Fulfillment,* perhaps you thought it was going to be all about how to have great sex. Well it is, but probably not the kind you were expecting. I hope that you've been pleasantly surprised as you learned about the things holding you back from true sexual intimacy. But now that you've learned how *not* to undermine your sexual and emotional fulfillment, let's talk about some specific ways to achieve it in your marriage.

INSPIRE—DON'T REQUIRE—INTIMACY

When my son was a toddler, he would often bring his toys and sit beside me to play. Regardless of what I was doing, he wanted to be near me. I found this very precious. But I also recall the many times that he would reach up to my cheek with his little hand and push my face toward something and say, "Wook, Mommy, wook!" I found this very annoying. Had he merely asked me to look, I would have been delighted. But because he felt the need to force me to look, the last thing I wanted to do was respond to his demand.

Fortunately, my son has outgrown this habit. Unfortunately, many wives have not. We still want our husbands to look inside of us, to pay attention to us, and to give us the emotional intimacy we crave, and we often try to force them to do so. When we attempt to require intimacy in this way, the last thing they want to do is respond to our demands (or manipulations, or however we choose to pursue it). However, there is a better way.

Imagine wanting to give a squirrel a nut. How would you do it? Would you chase the squirrel around the yard, grab him by his scrawny neck, and force the nut into his chubby cheeks? Of course not. You cannot require a squirrel to take a nut from you. However, you can inspire the squirrel to do this by simply placing a nut in your open palm, lying down beneath a tree, and falling asleep. When it's the squirrel's idea to take the nut, he'll do it.

Communicating intimately with our husbands is very similar to giving a squirrel a nut. Requiring it is futile. Intimacy can, however, be inspired. I used to go to bed expecting that my husband would talk with me for a while, not just about superficial stuff, but really engage in deep conversation. Even though I had heard psychologists explain that a man is capable of speaking only so many words each day and that they are almost all used up by the time he gets home from work, I thought I could drag it out of him. Needless to say, I usually went to sleep disappointed. Sometimes I went to sleep devastated, as I was trying to carry on a meaningful conversation and the only response I ultimately got once I stopped talking was "Zzzzzzzzzz."

Then I heard about this squirrel-and-nut theory and decided I may as well test it. I would go to bed with my husband at a decent hour, but rather than expecting to talk, I would simply say goodnight and allow him to drift off to sleep. After a few nights of this, Greg asked, "Are you upset with me about something?"

"No, why do you ask?" I replied.

"You've just been awfully quiet lately," he explained.

I smiled and said, "I'm not trying to give you the silent treatment, honey. I just know you are tired at night after a long day at work, and I want you to get plenty of rest."

Later that same night, we were getting in bed when Greg began asking me about my day and what I planned to do tomorrow. I responded, but didn't elaborate a great deal. Surprisingly, he kept asking more questions. Then he began telling me about some of the things that he'd had on his mind lately, asking me questions about what I think. We wound up talking for over an hour, and then moved closer to each other to lie in each other's arms. We decided to pray together, and by the time Greg finished praying, my desire to give him my body was positively overwhelming! Did he mind staying up a few more minutes to receive the gift I longed to give him? Absolutely not!

We stumbled onto something that night many years ago that we've never forgotten: True sexual fulfillment comes not just from a physical connection, but from an intimate mental, emotional, and spiritual connection as well. Although some nights we both drift off without much being said simply because we are both so tired, we have many nights when these intimate, brain-picking, heart-rendering, soul-searching conversations take place spontaneously. Sex doesn't always follow, but when it does, it's an incredibly fulfilling experience because the passion between us has been inspired, not required.

SERVE YOUR SPOUSE AS IF HE'S YOUR BEST FRIEND

If you choose to test this squirrel-and-nut theory yourself, please understand that it's not intended to be another manipulation game. By letting go of your expectations for your husband to meet your emotional needs and redirecting your focus on meeting his needs instead (whether those needs be for plenty of sleep or for physical pleasure), you are serving him. In this way, his desire will eventually be to serve you as well. He'll recognize your desire to meet his needs and that desire will be contagious if you do not abort the process by becoming impatient or expecting too much too soon. Just like intimacy, wholehearted service is inspired, not required.

When I speak of serving your husband, I'm not referring to the kind of serving you do in tennis, where you hit the ball to him and then claim, "Hey, the ball's in your court! It's your turn to serve me!" I'm referring to serving your husband's needs out of deep love and committed friendship, with no hidden motive and expecting nothing in return. Jesus referred to this type of service in the following passage:

> My command is this: Love each other as I have loved you. Greater love
> has no one than this, that [she] lay down [her] life for [her] friends.
> (John 15:12-13)

Ask yourself, "Do I consider my husband my friend?" I confess that I was guilty of not treating my husband as respectfully as I would a friend. I prided myself on being more verbal than he is, and I could win any argument hands down. When my husband told me, "You would have made a great lawyer," I thought his comment was a reflection of my intellect, but his comment was no compliment. He was right about one thing: I certainly never lost an argument. But I lost something far more important—*true intimacy with the man I love.*

Fortunately, Greg recognized that this "win my case at all cost" attitude was affecting our relationship, and he lovingly called me on it one day. I was arguing with him rather sarcastically. Then he asked me sincerely, "Shannon, would you talk to your best friend the way you are talking to me right now?" Ouch. I was expecting my husband to take everything I was dishing out, not realizing that he deserves best-friend treatment and common courtesy as much if not more so than anyone else in my life. I had been like Jekyll and Hyde—oozing smiles and sweetness to everyone outside our home while venting my frustrations on those within it. I've since come to realize that who I really am isn't the Shannon the world sees, but the person my family sees. Keeping this in mind has helped me act lovingly to my husband and children more consistently and has been like water and sunshine to help intimacy in our marriage blossom to its full potential.

Keep in mind that treating your husband like your best friend means treating him as the grown man that he is rather than as a child. Earlier in our marriage I often talked to Greg like he was a child, treating him as I would someone I had authority over. Rather than asking him politely to do something, I expected or even demanded it as a parent might expect a child to obey a command. I would complain about how he was dressed and pick out alternative clothes for him when there was nothing wrong with what he was wearing, commenting cleverly about "letting mother dress you." I even corrected his table manners in front of the children.

This mother-son dynamic can kill the desire for intimacy. *Men don't want to have sex with their mothers.* Your husband didn't marry you so he could have another mother, but so he could have a best friend. If you treat him like the grown man he is, you will foster in him an attitude of mutual respect, appreciation, and sexual desire toward you.

LEARN EACH OTHER'S LOVE LANGUAGE

As you make every effort to speak respectfully to your husband as your best friend and as the adult man that he is, you may recognize how much more loving you feel toward him when you talk to him. You may also feel as if the scales of communication are tipping out of balance when he doesn't reciprocate verbally to the level of your expectations, which brings us to another way to nurture intimacy: learning each other's love language.

As I mentioned earlier, most men speak fewer words than women speak. But that doesn't mean they don't communicate—they simply communicate in different ways. If we don't understand this, we may fail to pick up on what our husbands are telling us. Although I've had multiple experiences with such failure, one in particular stands out in my mind. We had been married one year and I often mailed cards from my office to Greg's. Every other month I would spend one of my lunch hours at the Hallmark store, stocking up on all kinds of sincere, clever, or hilariously funny greeting cards to say, "I love you!"

However, not long after our one-year anniversary, I noticed that I had never received a card from Greg. Not one. Not even a sticky note. I felt so neglected and furious over all the time and money I had spent picking out all these special cards, when there had been no reciprocation at all. Rather than ask why, I stopped sending cards, gave him the silent treatment, and withdrew emotionally (as if this were going to inspire him to send me a note of appreciation!).

I fumed for several days until I finally blew my top while standing in the

kitchen crying into my tuna salad. "In case you haven't noticed, I've stopped sending you cards each week! You've never once sent me a card! Do you know how
much that hurts? Or do you even care?"

My outburst shocked Greg, who waited until my screaming silenced to softly
respond, "But I mow your yard each week…and I wash your car…and I…"

"Well of course you do those things," I interrupted, "You live here too! Those
are your responsibilities!"

"But I do them out of love for you, Shannon!"

I wasn't convinced until Greg brought home the book I mentioned in chapter 6, *The Five Love Languages* by Gary Chapman. We read the book together
and I realized that Greg was right. "Acts of service" is a legitimate love language
and although it isn't my primary love language (mine is gifts), it is Greg's primary
way of expressing love to me. I also learned that the same way Greg's acts of service didn't fill my love tank, my Hallmark cards weren't really floating his boat
either. Our love languages are opposite each other—his highest (acts of service
and physical touch) are my lowest, and my highest (gifts and words of affirmation) are his lowest. We've had to be very intentional about speaking and understanding the other person's love language so that we can recognize each other's
loving expressions.

One anniversary not long afterward, Greg gave me a gift that I will never forget. It was a Hallmark card (finally!), but this one was full of hundreds of little pink
squares of paper. At first I thought this was his meager attempt at surprising me
with homemade confetti, but as I read the card, it touched me far more deeply
than confetti ever could. It read:

Shannon, I know that I don't do near as good of a job expressing my love to
you as you want me to. I'm not making any excuses, but my one desire is to
be able to recognize when you need affirmation of my love without you having to feel neglected or angry.

So I'm giving you all these slips of paper and asking you to please drop
one where I'll see it whenever I'm falling down on the job of making you feel
as special as you really are to me. Whenever I see a little pink slip of paper, I'll

be reminded of your need for me to express my love and commitment to you. Hopefully there are enough slips to get us through this lifetime, but if not, I'll cut some more.

Your loving husband, Greg

I think I've only resorted to planting a pink slip of paper in Greg's car twice in all the years since he did this. Just knowing how Greg wants to meet my emotional needs keeps my love tank full, whether he's been speaking my love language or not. And I've learned that if I want to express my love for him, I just do his laundry or weed the flower bed instead of driving to the Hallmark store.

As we learn to speak each other's love language, our love tanks are filled and we protect our marriage relationships from outside physical or emotional temptations. When either or both partners fail to recognize and meet the needs of their mate, these temptations can become overwhelming. I frequently hear women say (and have said it myself), "I'm so tempted because he doesn't meet my emotional needs!" But before you take aim at your husband for not meeting your emotional needs, look into your own emotional mirror and answer these questions:

- Do you know exactly what your emotional needs are yourself? (Many women don't; they just know they aren't fulfilled.) Do you know your own love language? (If not, I highly recommend that you read *The Five Love Languages*.)
- Have you lovingly and respectfully explained exactly what these needs are and how your husband can fill your love tank?
- Have you inspired him to try to understand your needs for emotional intimacy, or is this something you've attempted to require of him?
- How consistent have you been in meeting his physical needs (not just on special occasions, but according to his needs cycle)? Have you served his needs wholeheartedly and with a positive attitude?

Sheila shares this via e-mail to encourage women to recognize their unique role as their husband's sole source of pleasure:

If I don't cook for my husband, he can go to McDonald's. If I don't clean, he can hire a housekeeper. But if I don't respond to him physically, where can he go? Likewise, if my husband doesn't meet my emotional needs, I certainly can't go to another man. I am not supposed to be filled up with another man's compliments and attention. If we truly follow God's principles, die to ourselves, and serve each other, marriage could be a beautiful blessing!

While Sheila's word of wisdom is a valuable one, let me interject a disclaimer. I realize that some women have tried everything, including catering to their husband's physical needs, in an effort to wake him up emotionally. If this is you, and the above questions have only frustrated you rather than inspired you to try a new approach, then perhaps you both need to look into an emotional mirror with the help of a Christian counselor. If so, I encourage you to pursue healing as a couple.

While I can't promise you miraculous change, I can promise you that God sees the desires of your heart for intimacy and will honor your faithfulness. I can also promise that no relationship is beyond repair when two people begin serving each other unselfishly. I've seen many men get a revelation of their wives' emotional needs even after years of confusion and chaos in their marriage. If your husband needs a revelation such as this, remember these three points:

1. *Revelation doesn't come through human means but through divine means.* If you want your husband to seek to understand your innermost needs for his attention and affection, then pray that God would reveal this to him in His own time and in His own way. Then trust that God will do just that. Don't pester him, just pray for him. Leave the rest to God.

2. When you pray for your marriage relationship to improve, don't just pray for him. It takes two to tango. If your heart has become bitter or resentful of your husband's lack of sensitivity to your emotional needs, *pray for God to help you get your heart in the right place to inspire improvement.*

3. *Make every attempt to satisfy his sexual needs.* Don't just give in when he initiates, but take the initiative yourself to fulfill his innermost desires. Learn to give him the look that says, "You don't even have to ask! Take me now!" When you demonstrate that his needs are important to you, you may be surprised by how important your needs become to him.

UNDERSTAND THAT SEX IS A FORM OF WORSHIP

God designed sex to be shared between two bodies, two minds, two hearts, and two spirits which unite together to become a one-flesh union. If you've never experienced this one-flesh union in your marriage, then you are missing out on one of the most earth-shattering and fulfilling moments of your life!

So how can you move from having "just sex" to experiencing a form of lovemaking that satisfies every fiber of your being? By understanding that sex is actually a form of worshiping God that a husband and wife enter into together. When two become one flesh physically, mentally, emotionally, and spiritually, they are saying to God, "Your plan for our sexual and emotional fulfillment is a good plan. We choose your plan instead of our own."

Perhaps this passage from Mike Mason's *The Mystery of Marriage* will help you understand what God intended the honeymoon night and all other sexual encounters to be:

> What moment in a man's life can compare with that of the wedding night,
> when a beautiful woman takes off all her clothes and lies next to him in bed,
> and that woman is his wife? What can equal the surprise of finding out that
> the one thing above all others which mankind has been most enterprising
> and proficient in dragging through the dirt turns out in fact to be the most
> innocent thing in the world? Is there any other activity at all which an adult
> man and woman may engage in together (apart from worship) that is actu-
> ally more childlike, more clean and pure, more natural and wholesome and
> unequivocally right than is the act of making love? For if worship is the
> deepest available form of communion with God (and especially that
> particular act of worship known as Communion), then surely sex is the
> deepest communion that is possible between human beings, and as such
> is something absolutely essential (in more than a biological way) to our
> survival.[1]

For help in seeing your lovemaking as an act of worship, I suggest you begin by getting spiritually naked. Pray together and invite God into your bedroom to help you experience the joy and the wonder of what He created and gave you as a gift for marriage. If you are not in the habit of praying together as a couple already, this may seem awkward for you. If so, start by praying together each night with no intention of engaging in sex afterward.

As you talk and share openly with God and with each other, you will more than likely experience a spiritual closeness over time that may awaken your desire for a more intimate physical closeness. If so, you are moving in the right direction. As you both begin to experience this greater level of spiritual connection (and assuming you remain faithful in keeping your mind focused on intimacy only with your husband rather than with another), you will discover a deeper level of emotional fulfillment in your relationship. For a woman, it is these deeper levels of mental, emotional, and spiritual intimacy which are key to igniting a passion for physical intimacy with your husband.

Once a woman experiences the intimacy of being mentally, emotionally, and spiritually naked before her husband and feeling as if she is loved for who she truly is on the inside, her natural response will be to want to give the outside package physically to her admirer. Notice I said *want to,* not *feel that she has to.* Our desire to give our bodies as a trophy to the man who has captivated our hearts and committed his faithfulness to us sets the stage for genuine sexual fulfillment. Sex performed merely out of obligation or duty will never satisfy you (or him) like presenting your passion-filled mind, body, heart, and soul to your husband on a silver platter, inviting your lover to come into your garden and taste its choice fruits (see Song of Songs 4:16).

CULTIVATE GENUINE INTIMACY IN YOUR LOVEMAKING

In order to maximize fulfillment in your marriage, consider implementing these practical dos and don'ts for cultivating genuine intimacy in your lovemaking:

- *Be prepared for anything* by making feminine hygiene a daily routine. Nothing will keep you from feeling the freedom to engage in spontaneous physical intimacy faster than unshaven legs or a feeling of personal unclean-liness. Shave your legs as often as possible and cleanse your genital area daily with a mild soap such as Summer's Eve Intimate Cleanser. Mak-ing feminine hygiene as much a part of your morning or evening routine as brushing your teeth will go a long way in giving you the confidence to pursue sexual fulfillment anytime you feel the desire to engage in physical intimacy.

- *Keep a dim light on* and open your eyes often while making love. You don't turn off the lights and close your eyes to feel more intimate conversing with a friend, do you? My experience has been that when it's dark or when I keep my eyes closed, I'm far more tempted to allow my mind to wander into someone else's arms. Making frequent visual contact with my husband keeps me focused on him and keeps my thoughts in the pleasurable experi-ences of the present, which certainly adds to my sexual fulfillment. Drink in the beauty of you and your husband engaged in the act of pleasuring each other sexually and enjoy the view.

- *Train your brain to focus* strictly on your husband during sex. Some women have had so many sexual experiences with other men that they find physi-cal intimacy with their husband difficult to concentrate on or even boring. What a pity that we've learned to mistake intensity for intimacy. While you may think being sexual with a stranger would be more exciting, it certainly wouldn't be intimate at all, and that is what women truly crave. Intimacy occurs only as a result of knowing each other inside and out. You aren't going to fully experience that with a stranger, but only with the man you live and grow old with. If you need to train your mind to focus on your husband during sex, try meditating on the word *husband* or *worship*. Remind yourself frequently, "This is my husband. Pleasuring him sexually is an act of worship to God." Even pray during your sexual moments that God would maximize your intimacy by helping you to focus exclusively on each other.

- *Be open to discussing* ways that your husband can enhance your physical pleasure and inquire about the same for him. Often we know our own bodies and what feels good far better than we know the opposite sex's body, and most men are very open to learning all they can about the fascinating area that is intended exclusively for his pleasure. Also feel free to discuss sexual fantasies with each other, as long as those fantasies involve no one other than the two of you. Remember, a woman is most aroused by what she hears, and sensual words spoken between the two of you while engaging in physical intimacy can cause a woman to melt like butter.

- *Don't cave in* to the idea that it's okay to entertain any inappropriate thought so you can reach orgasm more quickly. Just because it takes most women approximately five to ten times longer to orgasm as it does men doesn't mean we should just throw caution to the wind and get it over with for the sake of time. There's something more valuable at stake here than time, and that is ultimate sexual fulfillment as God intended it. Your husband won't be offended by how long it takes you to orgasm if he knows you are focusing strictly on him and the pleasure he is providing you. You can retrain your brain to avoid inappropriate places and concentrate on keeping the home fires burning.

- *Don't keep score* as to how many times each of you gets to orgasm. One friend confided, "I told my husband that my orgasm is just as important as his and that I refuse to have sex unless he is going to invest the time and energy into my orgasm as well." Instead of her experiencing orgasm as often as he wanted to, he only experienced it as often as she needed to, which wasn't all that often. Several months later she was devastated over the feelings of resentment in their relationship and realized that requiring fair play in their sex life was a bit unfair. Your marital relationship is designed by God so that you can complete each other, not compete with each other. If he needs a sexual release and you don't, providing a quick fix (also known as "a quickie") will show that you aren't a scorekeeper but a cooperative team player. Such sensitivity to his needs will cause him to be your biggest fan.

- *Don't hide your body* from your husband thinking you don't measure up to the latest fashion models. Most men really don't care about that. What they do care about, however, is the enjoyment of taking their wife in through their eyes, knowing that this is sacred property belonging solely to them. Randy tells of his discovery of the beauty of his wife:

> Thinking that maybe [all the sexual gratification I was collecting through my eyes] was why I'd lost my appetite for [my wife] Regina, I began starving my eyes. I couldn't believe what happened! Regina is no longer just a friend. She's become a goddess, at least to me. And it's funny—the more I draw only from her, the more my tastes change. Those little rolls of fat on her back and sides used to bother me. Now, as I run my finger over them, they actually turn me on. Isn't that crazy? And that little bit of rear end that hangs below her underwear? Before, it only emphasized to me how much weight she'd gained. Now, that little piece just explodes my desire for her. Regina may not be a supermodel, but I'm no day at the beach either. Yet to me, she's like Miss America now.[2]

Let me warn you that when you experience sexual fulfillment on this deep level (not just a physical level, but also a mental, emotional, and spiritual level as well), you may notice some strange occurrences. Because of the deep emotional release that experiencing an orgasm can be for a woman, you may find yourself bursting into tears in his arms afterward. Or you may begin laughing hysterically (not *at* your husband, but *with* your husband). Perhaps you will be motivated to put on some worship music and worship together, just the two of you in your bedroom. You just never know how you are going to be inspired to react when you feel so incredibly fulfilled from the top of your head to the bottom of your toes and all points in between (including your mind, heart, and spirit, of course). You may even find yourself enjoying and initiating sex more often than your husband does!

REBUILDING ON A FIRM FOUNDATION

Before we close this chapter on discovering a new level of intimacy with your husband, I want to address one final issue. Some of you may wish that you had learned these principles years ago, because it may have kept you from engaging in a physical or emotional affair. Now that you're trying to become a woman of sexual and emotional integrity, you wonder what effect your secret would have on your marriage if you were to tell your husband about it.

Some psychologists say, "There's no reason for your partner to know about your affair. What purpose does it serve to clear your conscience if it is only going to upset him?" I am all for protecting someone else's feelings by not burdening him with unnecessary information. I also understand your commitment to keeping your marriage together, especially if you feel that divulging your secrets would drive the nail into your marriage coffin. However, before you decide you would never confess an affair to your husband, ask yourself these questions:

- Is harboring these secrets ultimately as damaging to our marriage as what I did in the first place?
- Am I robbing myself and my husband of true intimacy and sexual fulfillment because of the guilt I wrestle with?
- Is my confidence that my husband loves me based on who he thinks I am—a wife who has never betrayed him?

If the answer to these questions is yes, I encourage you to look at this issue in a different light. Discovering a new level of intimacy in your marriage may be very difficult if you can't let your husband see completely into you. As I mentioned previously, intimacy can best be understood by breaking the word down into syllables: *in-to-me-see.* Marital secrets serve no purpose but to alienate you from the only one who can provide the level of intimacy you truly desire as a sexual being. If you keep secrets from each other, you may build a wall between you and ultimate sexual and emotional fulfillment.

However, through humble confession and eventual restoration of trust, you can turn those walls into bridges that will bring the two of you closer together than ever before. I believe you can rebuild on a firmer foundation by opening up to your husband, confessing your sin, seeking healing counsel, and recruiting his help to overcome future temptations. After all, when you believe your husband loves you for who he thinks you are (yet you see yourself as a different person because you know things he doesn't), that's not intimate nor is it fulfilling.

James 5:16 says, "Therefore confess your sins to each other and pray for each other so that you may be healed." Obviously James felt that confession is good for the soul. While it may be dreadfully painful at first, I believe confession is ultimately good for the marriage as well.

Perhaps your honesty will create an environment where he finally feels safe to discuss his innermost sexual struggles. Make a pact that you won't judge him for how he is prone to visual stimulation and that he won't judge you for how you are prone to emotional stimulation. Your unconditional love can inspire him to guard his eyes, and his unconditional love can inspire you to guard your heart. So consider taking off the mask and allowing him to see the good, the bad, and the ugly. And don't cringe when he, too, takes his mask off. Remember, we are all human beings with our own unique struggles. Your marriage can be a place where you and your spouse can sharpen each other with accountability, not stab each other with judgment.

In addition, if you struggle sexually because of abuse you have experienced in your past, tell your husband what happened to you. When Greg and I were first married, I didn't really want to talk about how my uncles had attempted to molest me as a young teenager. I was afraid he would view me as "damaged goods" and not be as drawn to me sexually. However, my counselor encouraged me to discuss these fears with Greg, and although it was uncomfortable, we made a huge breakthrough as a result of the conversation. I told him how one of my uncles would wake me up in the middle of the night to come into the living room so he could kiss me while his wife was sleeping. I mentioned how sometimes I could still smell the smoke on his breath and feel his bushy mustache tickling my lip, a feeling that made my insides flip-flop with disgust. I felt very ashamed even saying the words, somehow feeling as if this was my fault instead of my uncle's.

But Greg was busy making connections and discerning how he could help me heal from these wounds. He compassionately responded, "Could that be why you don't like it when I wake you up in the middle of the night to hug and kiss you?" Although I had never made that connection before, I had to confess that I didn't like to be startled with physical affection, especially in the middle of the

Intimacy Busters	Intimacy Boosters
1. having sex as a means of closeness	1. having sex as a response to closeness
2. requiring intimacy from your spouse	2. inspiring intimacy with your spouse
3. expecting your needs to be served	3. serving each other's needs
4. sarcastic or condescending talk	4. conversing respectfully as best friends
5. treating him like your child	5. treating him like your husband
6. hiding thoughts and fantasies	6. offering mental nakedness
7. making unhealthy comparisons of your husband or yourself	7. accepting each other unconditionally
8. failing to use each other's love language	8. learning and speaking each other's love language
9. assuming he should need a sexual release only as often as you do	9. willing to satisfy his sexual needs according to his needs cycle
10. pestering him to change his ways or giving him the silent treatment	10. praying for and with each other consistently
11. considering sex a worldly act	11. considering sex an act of worship
12. giving into sex out of obligation	12. initiating sex out of passionate love
13. feeling personally unclean	13. maintaining feminine hygiene
14. darkening the room or closing eyes during sex	14. engaging visually in sexual activity
15. expressing frustration that he's "not doing it right"	15. discussing what brings you pleasure
16. trying to rush orgasm by entertaining inappropriate thoughts	16. savoring sexual intimacy without pressure to get it over with
17. requiring orgasm as often as he ejaculates	17. refraining from keeping score in the bedroom
18. masturbating without your spouse present or involved	18. depending totally on each other for sexual pleasure
19. showing body shame and extreme inhibition	19. stimulating visually with nakedness
20. harboring secrets of moral failure or sexual abuse	20. remaining open and honest about sexual struggles and fears

Figure 10.1

night. This was a great relief to Greg, as he had always taken my lack of response as disinterest in him. Greg also asked, "Is this why you don't kiss me near as often since I've grown a mustache?" Once again, I felt as if he hit the nail on the head. The very next morning, Greg shaved his face completely clean, and we spent half an hour catching up on all the kisses that mustache had unknowingly robbed us of.

When we allow the person who is most committed to loving us unconditionally to see what is truly on the inside of us, regardless of how ashamed or broken we feel over it, the rewards are endless. We can gain confidence and courage, experience healing of painful memories, and enjoy genuine intimacy with the person we love and trust the most.

KEEPING FOXES OUT OF THE VINEYARD

This passage in Song of Songs has often caught my eye:

> Catch for us the foxes,
>   the little foxes
> that ruin the vineyards,
>   our vineyards that are in bloom. (2:15)

The vineyard is a metaphor for the relationship shared between lovers. I believe a fully blossoming vineyard symbolizes a relationship in which mental, emotional, spiritual, and physical intimacy is at its peak. But I've often wondered what the foxes that ruin the vineyard are a symbol of.

As I thought and prayed about this, I began to recall the many things in our marriage which were like foxes ruining our vineyard, creating distance rather than intimacy in my marriage. Greg and I have worked to recognize these "intimacy busters" and turn them around to become "intimacy boosters." The list on page 159 sums up many of the principles we've been talking about in this chapter.

As you cultivate genuine intimacy with your husband by avoiding the intimacy busters and enjoying the intimacy boosters, you will experience the kind of mental, emotional, spiritual, and physical pleasure that God intends for your marriage relationship.

Let him kiss me with the kisses of his mouth—
     for your love is more delightful than wine....

My lover is to me a sachet of myrrh
     resting between my breasts....

How handsome you are, my lover!
     Oh, how charming!
     And our bed is verdant....

Like an apple tree among the trees of the forest
     is my lover among the young men.
I delight to sit in his shade,
     and his fruit is sweet to my taste.
He has taken me to the banquet hall,
     and his banner over me is love....

Awake, north wind,
     and come, south wind!
Blow on my garden,
     that its fragrance may spread abroad.

Let my lover come into his garden
     and taste its choice fruits....

His mouth is sweetness itself;
     he is altogether lovely.
This is my lover, this my friend....

I belong to my lover,
     and his desire is for me.
          —Song of Songs 1:2,13,16; 2:3-4; 4:16; 5:16; 7:10

retreating with the Lord

I am my beloved's and my beloved is mine.

SONG OF SOLOMON 6:3 (NRSV)

A radiant bride greeted her guests with a brilliant smile as she entered the reception hall after the wedding ceremony. She gracefully moved and milled about the room, the train of her stunning white gown flowing along the floor behind her, her veil cascading down her button-adorned back.

She conversed with each guest one by one, taking the time to mingle and soak up the compliments. "You look absolutely lovely." "Your dress is divine." "I've never seen a more beautiful bride." "What a stunning ceremony." The lavish praises rang on and on. The bride couldn't be more proud or more appreciative of the crowd's adoration. She could have listened to them swoon over her all evening. As a matter of fact, she did.

But where was the groom? All the attention focused on the bride and never once did she call anyone's attention to her husband. She didn't even notice his absence at her side. Scanning the room, I searched for him, wondering, "Where could he be?"

I finally found him, but not where I expected him to be. The groom stood alone over in the corner of the room with his head down. As he stared at his ring, twisting the gold band that had just been placed on his finger by his bride, tears trickled down his cheeks and onto his hands. That is when I noticed the nail scars. The groom was Jesus.

He waited, but the bride never once turned her face toward her groom. She never held His hand. She never introduced the guests to Him. She operated independently of Him.

I awoke from my dream with a sick feeling in my stomach. "Lord, is this how I made you feel when I was looking for love in all the wrong places?" I wept at the thought of hurting Him so deeply.

Unfortunately, this dream illustrates exactly what is happening between God and millions of His people. He betroths Himself to us, we take His name (as "Christians"), and then we go about our lives looking for love, attention, and affection from every source under the sun except from the Son of God, the Lover of our souls.

Oh, how Jesus longs for His own to acknowledge Him, to introduce Him to our friends, to withdraw to be alone with Him, to cling to Him for our identity, to gaze longingly into His eyes, to love Him with all our heart and soul.

What about you? Do you have this kind of love relationship with Christ? Do you experience the inexplicable joy of intimacy with the One who loves you with a passion far deeper, far greater than anything you could find here on earth? I know from experience that you can.

HOW DO I GET THERE FROM HERE?

Maybe you are wondering how to get from where you are now to this much deeper, more gratifying level of intimacy with Jesus Christ. It would help to look at where our spiritual journey begins as believers and how our relationship with God evolves as we travel down the path toward spiritual maturity. Life coach and international lecturer Jack Hill (www.royal-quest.com) explains that there are six progressive levels of relationship with God, as found in the following metaphors in scripture:

- potter/clay relationship
- shepherd/sheep relationship
- master/servant relationship
- friend/friend relationship
- father/daughter relationship
- groom/bride relationship

I believe God gave us these metaphors to increase our understanding of His many-faceted personality and to help us comprehend the depth of His perfect love for us (although the human mind can not fathom such depth). These metaphors illustrate the maturing of our love relationship with God. Just as children develop physically until they reach adulthood, believers in Christ develop spiritually in stages as we walk down the road to spiritual maturity. As we examine the dynamics of each of these stages, perhaps you can discern what level of intimacy you are currently experiencing in your walk with God. You can also determine what level of connection you can anticipate as your relationship with God continues to blossom.

POTTER/CLAY RELATIONSHIP

When we first come to Christ, our spiritual life has little shape or form. We submit ourselves to Jesus Christ as our Savior and ask God to begin shaping us into what He wants us to be. "We are the clay, you are the potter; we are all the work of your hand" (Isaiah 64:8; see also Jeremiah 18:4-6). As a piece of clay, we can allow ourselves to be molded and become a product of the Potter who cares for us, but we cannot express our love back to Him. We can't experience any deep sense of intimacy if we remain in this level of relationship. Why? Because a lump of clay's value is based on how it can be used. When we comply and feel God using us, we feel good about ourselves. When we mess up or don't have a clear sense of purpose, we feel guilty and distant from God. We often withdraw because we believe He is angry with us due to our poor performance. Ephesians 2:10 says, "For we are God's workmanship, created in Christ Jesus to do good works, which God prepared in advance for us to do." This scripture affirms that it is important for us to submit to God and allow Him to shape our lives into something that brings Him honor. However, He doesn't want our relationship to stagnate there. He wants it to continue growing in depth and intimacy.

SHEPHERD/SHEEP RELATIONSHIP

It may not be flattering to be compared to sheep, but this metaphor illustrates how well God takes care of His people, just as a shepherd carefully tends his flock. God spoke through the prophet Ezekiel:

For this is what the Sovereign LORD says: I myself will search for my sheep and look after them. As a shepherd looks after his scattered flock when he is with them, so will I look after my sheep. I will rescue them from all the places where they were scattered.... They will lie down in good grazing land, and there they will feed in a rich pasture on the mountains of Israel. I myself will tend my sheep and have them lie down, declares the Sovereign LORD. (34:11-15; see also the parable of the good shepherd in John 10:1-18).

Although sheep know the shepherd's voice and will follow him, they have no idea what the heart of the shepherd feels for them. Sheep are unable to share the shepherd's dreams and hopes. They are merely concerned with their daily need for food and water. While it is important for us to follow and trust God as our care-taker and provider just as a sheep follows a shepherd, God longs for us to have far more with Him.

MASTER/SERVANT RELATIONSHIP

While sheep stay outside, servants at least live in the same household as the master and can talk with him, as long as it is business. The servant enjoys a more intimate relationship. This level of relationship is referred to in the parable of the talents (Matthew 25:14-30) and in the parable of the ten minas (Luke 19:11-27). How-ever, servants know little of what is happening with the master other than what they are directly involved with. A servant's value is based on how well she can com-plete the master's will. If she does not comply according to her master's expecta-tions, she will be removed from the household and replaced by another. While it is important for us to serve God wholeheartedly and do His will, God still longs to have an even greater level of intimacy with us than this.

FRIEND/FRIEND RELATIONSHIP

A servant's relationship with his master is based on business and performance, while love and mutual concern is the basis for a friend's relationship with another friend. Jesus spoke very clearly to His disciples about this deeper level of intimacy that He shared with them when He said, "I no longer call you servants, because a servant does not know his master's [personal] business. Instead, I have called you friends, for everything that I learned from my Father I have made known to you" (John 15:15). Jesus is saying, "I value you, not just because of how you serve me, but because you share my heart." A friend's value lies not so much in what she does, but in who she is as a personal confidant. God wants to be our friend, and He wants us as His friend. We can experience this friendship level of intimacy, as James 2:23 tells us, "And the scripture was fulfilled that says, 'Abraham believed God, and it was credited to him as righteousness,' and he was called God's friend." Also, Proverbs 22:11 says, "[She] who loves a pure heart and whose speech is gracious will have the king for [her] friend."

Yet even as close as two friends can be, blood runs thicker than water.

FATHER/DAUGHTER RELATIONSHIP

As we realize and accept the truth that we are not just God's lump of clay, sheep, servant, or even friend, but also God's very own child, we can experience tremendous healing from childhood wounds and disappointments. We can allow God to be the Father or the Mother (He possesses qualities of both genders) that we so desperately need or want. We can be freed from the burden of trying to perform or produce for Him when we understand that He loves us not for what we do, but because of who we are as His daughters. Paul wrote:

> But when the time had fully come, God sent his Son, born of a woman,
> born under law, to redeem those under law, that we might receive the full
> rights of [daughters]. Because you are [daughters], God sent the Spirit of
> his Son into our hearts, the Spirit who calls out, "Abba, Father." (Galatians
> 4:4-6)

As wonderful and healing as the father/child relationship is, the groom/bride relationship promises the most intimate connection of all.

GROOM/BRIDE RELATIONSHIP

Once a woman becomes a bride, the focus of her life and priorities change and all other people and priorities pale in comparison to this primary love relationship. Again, this metaphor illustrates a much deeper truth—God desires a level of relationship with us such that we are deeply in love with Him, that we delight to simply be in His presence, that we know Him personally both publicly and privately, and that our focus and priorities become aligned with His desires.

Perhaps you feel that you can relate to God as our Father, Savior, or Lord but are struggling with the idea of relating to God as intimately as you would a husband. While some may even say that it is irreverent to relate to God in such an intimate way, God has always longed for this kind of relationship with His chosen people. He said through the prophet Hosea, "I will betroth you to me forever; I will betroth you in righteousness and justice, in love and compassion. I will betroth you in faithfulness and you will acknowledge the LORD" (2:19-20).

According to this passage God has extended an eternal commitment of love to us as His people, a love so deep, so wide, and so great that no earthly mind can possibly fathom it. It is the kind of gift that should inspire us to reciprocate with as equal of a gift of love as is humanly possible.

Scripture often refers to the church as the *bride* of Christ. If you have received Christ as Savior, you are His betrothed. John obviously understood God's desire to betroth us to Himself in this type of intimate bride-and-groom relationship. He writes:

Let us rejoice and be glad
  and give him glory!
For the wedding of the Lamb has come,
  and his bride has made herself ready.
Fine linen, bright and clean
  was given her to wear.
(Fine linen stands for the righteous acts of the saints.)

Then the angel said to me, "Write: 'Blessed are those who are invited to the wedding supper of the Lamb!'" And he added, "These are the true words of God." (Revelation 19:7-9)

What began as an engagement relationship between God and His own in the Garden of Eden will finally be consummated at the wedding supper of the Lamb when Jesus Christ returns to claim His bride (the church). In the last line of this scripture, the angel said specifically to add that these are God's "true words," as if the angel somehow knew that this type of bridal relationship with the Almighty would be difficult for us to fathom. But His bridegroom love for us is very real.

So how do we cultivate a bridal love for Jesus and enjoy this intimate relationship that He longs to have with us? By falling in love with Him and attempting to pursue Him as passionately as He has been pursuing us all along.

FALLING HEAD OVER HEELS IN LOVE

Christie, in her early twenties, began to hunger for a deeper, more meaningful time of fellowship with God. After praying for insight on how to satisfy this hunger, she decided to set one night apart each week to "date" Jesus. As bizarre as that may sound to you, Christie so looks forward to separating herself from work, school, and other friends to enjoy her Friday nights alone with Jesus.

Christie explains:

Sometimes I go to a park for a picnic and prayer night. Sometimes I read my Bible and write letters from God in my journal, including all the wisdom, correction, encouragement, and affirmation I sense Him giving to me. Sometimes I go to Barnes & Noble to drink coffee with the Lord and to read whatever book from the Christian Living section He guides me to.

Sometimes I cook a wonderful meal and set the table for two, talking to God as if He is actually sitting there at my table with me because I know that He is. Sometimes I sense His love so strongly that I feel giddy! One night I even set the table for four and invited God, Jesus, and the Holy Spirit to dine with me. I felt so overjoyed and affirmed by their presence. It felt like we were having a heavenly party!

If my roommate walked in during one of these dinner parties, she would probably think of having me committed to a mental institution! I guess I would tell her I'm already committed—to God! I love my precious time with the Lord, and if I skip a single week, I miss Him and I know He misses me!

WALKING AND TALKING WITH JESUS

Some women enjoy sitting in a comfy chair to meditate or for their quiet time with the Lord. Not me. I either get distracted thinking about all the things I should be doing or I get sleepy. I enjoy walking and talking with the Lord. I usually drop my children off at school and then drive to one of the many secluded country roads where I have a four-mile stretch measured off in my mind. I start by stretching and taking deep breaths, thanking God that He's given me another day to be alive and fully functioning. Drinking in the beauty of the towering trees, inhaling the aroma of wildflowers, feeling the breeze caress my face, I commune with God outdoors during my walk in a way I never could otherwise. As I walk, I talk to Him about five things:

- Adoration (telling Him all the wonderful things I love about Him, such as how His mercies are new every morning, His incomparable strength, His compassionate character, and so on)
- Confession (acknowledging the many ways I miss the mark and asking Him to reveal anything I've done or attitude that I've had that has caused Him to grieve)
- Thanksgiving (expressing my gratitude for the multitude of blessings in my life)
- Supplication (asking for a special blessing or His divine guidance in certain matters)
- Others (intercession for family and friends, women God has called me to serve, coworkers, and anyone else God brings to mind)

You might wonder, "How do you remember all that?" With the acronym ACTSO—Adoration, Confession, Thanksgiving, Supplication, and Others—I ACT by praying SO that I can feel connected to God. And His response is sometimes audible, not to my ears, but to my heart. As I confess, I often sense Him comforting me, saying, "It's okay. I'm not going to let that come between us." As I ask Him for guidance, He usually steers my mind toward a solution I hadn't thought of before. As I pray for others, He regularly prompts me to do or say something specifically for their benefit. This response time is a vital part of my prayer life. He already knows what is on my heart without my saying a word. I need to make time to listen to what is on His heart because without listening I'll never have a clue. God often reminds me of this as I am walking and rambling on and on. Sometimes by the time I reach the two- or three-mile mark on my four-mile hike, I'll sense God saying, "Remember to leave Me some time. I've got a lot I want to say to you today." Does this make me feel special that the God of the universe wants time to talk specifically with me each day? You bet. And He wants to talk with you each day as well. Is there a spot in your Day-Timer when you can give Him a standing (or walking) appointment?

Enoch walked with God for three hundred years, then God took him away (Genesis 5:21-24). He never tasted death. I can just imagine that Enoch's walk with God was so intimate, so joyous, that one day God simply said, "You know, Enoch, we are closer to my house than to yours. Let's just go to mine."

Don and Deyon Stephens, cofounders of Mercy Ships International, tell of Don's Aunt Lilly, who had a regular walking date with God at 4 P.M. every day. "If you were visiting and Aunt Lilly disappeared around four o'clock, you just knew where she was going and that she'd be back around five. She never allowed anything to keep her from her date with Jesus." Aunt Lilly died within the past few years, and when Don was preparing to preach her funeral, he inquired as to the exact time of her death. His suspicion was confirmed when the hospital stated her time of death as 4 P.M. Aunt Lilly didn't miss her walk with Jesus.

A RESTFUL RENDEZVOUS

When I am stressed or feeling overwhelmed, I have found that being still and resting in God's presence helps me cope with the demands of marriage, motherhood, and ministry. While I used to be too high-strung to slow down long enough to take these "sanity breaks" or not bother lying down unless I had two hours to nap, I now seize whatever time I can whenever I can. If I have twenty minutes before heading out the door to soccer practice, I let my kids know that I need some "Mommy time." I close the door, set the timer, lay down on my bed, and imagine Jesus holding me, stroking my cheek, even running His fingers through my hair. I often meditate on Psalm 46:10, "Be still, and know that I am God." These few minutes can alleviate stress, lift my spirits, adjust my attitude, and give me a second wind to continue going about my busy day. Just knowing that the almighty God sees how hard I am working to maintain a household, raise a family, and run a ministry and sensing His loving encouragement to press on gives me the strength to keep running the race, even when I'm stumbling or feel like quitting.

I don't know about you, but I desperately need that kind of encouragement and affirmation. I used to perform for others to get this need met. I knocked myself out for my boss, going way above and beyond the call of duty, just so I could hear, "You did a great job." I fixed myself up all the time, dressing to arouse men and hoping to hear, "Don't you look gorgeous today!" I went out of my way to do things for people just to hear them say, "I appreciate your thoughtfulness." But when you look to others for your affirmation, you have to find ways get a fresh supply, which eventually will run you ragged. But I have found that God's affirmation fills my emotional tank even more than any human's flattering words will. When I sense the God of the universe saying to me, "I see everything you are doing and your hard work brings me great joy.... You are so beautiful to me even when you are sleeping.... I see your heart and you are so very special to me," His sentiments send me reeling further than any man ever could.

RUNNING AWAY WITH THE LORD

In addition to putting aside some time each day to rest in the arms of God and converse with Jesus, I recommend that you schedule a sabbatical alone with God at least once or twice each year. Based on the word *Sabbath,* a sabbatical is an extended amount of time set apart for the further cultivation of a love relationship with Jesus. Again, God loves it when you honor Him with the gift of time. What better way to honor Him and your desire for His presence than to schedule an extended rendezvous with Him.

I've practiced sabbaticals over the past several years, and I've never experienced one where God didn't lavish life-renewing love on me and give me a major revelation for my life or my ministry to guide me. I remember one retreat where I went alone just to be with God and align my heart with His. I had just been granted a partial scholarship from a very prestigious college to work on a master's degree in counseling, plus my local church offered to cover the rest of the tuition and my books. I was blown away at this incredible opportunity, and it never crossed my mind that this wasn't a gift from God. However, on the second day of my retreat as I was thanking Him for this incredible provision, I sensed a heavy burden on His heart. "What could possibly be wrong?" I wondered. I continued to pray about it and just listen. "Are you trying to tell me something, God? Is there anything I'm not seeing here?"

In my mind's eye I saw a vision of a mama bird leaving two little baby birds in the nest. Then I realized I hadn't given as much thought to what this new endeavor would mean to my four-year-old daughter and one-year-old son. I began praying for my daughter and son and asking God to show me why I felt such a heavy burden about such a huge financial blessing.

Then I sensed God asking, "Do you trust me enough to lay these scholarships on the altar? Will you sacrifice them for the sake of my will for your family?" *Whoa.* I loved my family, but the thought of giving up over fifty thousand dollars of free tuition seemed almost idiotic. However, by the time I left to go home, I knew beyond a shadow of a doubt that this is exactly what God wanted me to do. As I walked through the door of my home, I hugged my children tightly and looked at my husband with tears in my eyes. "I'm giving up the scholarships," I said. "I'm not going back to school until the kids are much older. If God provided the money once, He can provide it again when the time is right. I know it's a shock, but I have a real peace that this is what God wants me to do."

"Then why are you crying?" Greg asked.

I responded, "Because I am so thankful to have these baby birds in our nest and God to guide me in raising them!"

Of course I had to explain that one to my husband, but I've never regretted that decision. I knew it was God's will even if it wasn't my own at the time. I knew the peace I felt about it was a gift from Him worth far more than any scholarship. And I knew that all things work together for the good of those who love God and are called according to His purpose—even for moms without a master's degree.

When I've asked women what hinders them from making the effort to run away for a retreat with the Lord, the three most common answers I received have been lack of time, lack of finances, and lack of help with the house and kids. If running away with God is something that you really want to do, you'll get creative enough to make it happen. For instance, if you feel you don't have a weekend for time alone with God, ask Him to show you ways to reprioritize to make some extended time available during the week, even if it's only a few hours. We all have the same twenty-four hours in a day, and He'll help you carve out time for such a high priority. If you can't afford to spend money, be creative about how to get some time away. I often ask some people in our church to use their lake house for a few days during the week, and I take my own food or I fast during those days.

If you feel you can't go away and retreat with the Lord because of household and parenting responsibilities, try explaining to your husband that you will be a much better wife and mommy if you have this time to yourself to spend with God. (My husband encourages me to go on these sabbaticals when I get out of sorts!) If you are a single mom and you cannot recruit sufficient assistance from other relatives, make a deal with a friend in a similar situation. Schedule two different weekends or other occasions when the two of you will swap houses. On the first weekend, you and your kids go to her house to keep her children and tend to her chores while she enjoys time alone with God at your house. Make it wonderful for her by putting wildflowers in a vase and some fresh fruit on the table. Stock the bathroom with bubble bath, some facial scrub, and a sweet-smelling candle. Leave a mint on the pillow and some relaxing CDs in the bedroom. Then when it is your turn, she'll take care of your house and kids and treat you to a getaway at her house with God.

While it's tempting to send your kids away and stay home, I have found that this never works as well because I get distracted by the mounds of laundry, rampant dust bunnies, and stacks of mail. So go somewhere. Offer to house-sit for people. If you are adventurous, go camping. Get away from the normal surroundings and routines and have a refreshing new experience with the Lord.

In case you are wondering, "What would I *do* on a retreat with God?" (that's the Martha in us all, feeling like we have to *do* something), here are some ideas to get your creative juices flowing. Remember, think like Mary (see Luke 10:38-42)! This is an incredible opportunity to get away from it all and bask in Jesus' presence, although some of these ideas will suit both the Mary (the worshiper) and the Martha (the busy doer) in you. Any of these ideas can be adapted to fit your schedule, whether you manage to carve out three days, one day, or only a few hours.

"Past, Present, and Future" Retreat

Break up your time into three segments. During the first segment, think about your childhood or recent past. Are there people you need to forgive? Are there people you need to ask forgiveness of? Take time to write letters to those people, clearing your conscience and speaking a blessing over them. Next, examine your present. Make a list of how you spend your time each day and see if you are investing in your true priorities or simply putting out fires day by day. Ask God to show you how to restructure your time each day to accomplish those things and invest in those relationships most important to you. Finally, focus on your future. What are your ultimate goals in life spiritually, relationally, professionally, and/or financially? Ask God to show you how to meet those goals and how to become the best steward possible of the precious time He's blessed you with here on earth.

Hobby Retreat

What do you enjoy doing most? Painting? Reading? Writing? Make some time to do just that alone with God. Whatever it is, pack up your tools or books or whatever you'll need and run away. Paint with passion, dedicating your masterpiece to the glory of God. Take a good Christian living or Christian fiction book and read voraciously without apology. Take a huge stack of index cards to jot down ideas and a laptop computer. Seek His direction and brainstorm things you could creatively write about that would glorify God.

"Prayer, Praise, and Pampering" Retreat

Too often we try to sit in His presence at 6 A.M., half-awake in our nightgowns, feeling anything but glamorous and passionate. Remember the painstaking process of getting ready for a hot date with that someone special? A process that we only wish we had time for in these "got to get myself and everyone else ready in forty-five minutes or less" days? Make time for a spiritual spa weekend. Take all of your favorite bath-and-beauty products and pamper yourself to go before the King. You'll be amazed at how, when you feel pretty on the outside, passion flows freely from the inside. Your heart of worship will soar and you won't want to stop talking with God, just like you could have conversed all night with that special date long ago. Although God certainly loves us even with unshaven legs, no makeup, and a bed-head hairdo, He also deserves to occasionally have His princess sit at His feet while she is looking and feeling her best.

Intercessor's Retreat

Many women have such a burden for others, but the burden of a busy schedule keeps us from praying until we feel a peace for those individuals. Take your Bible, your address book, some pretty stationery, and a pen, and run away for an extended time of intercession. Pray for those you are closest to and anyone else that God lays on your heart. Ask God to give you a special scripture to pass on to those individuals that you care so much about, and write it in a sweet note to them. Whether I am struggling, striving, surviving, or succeeding, it feels so good to get a note from a friend or family member saying, "You've been on my heart and I am praying for you." It feels even better to be the one to brighten someone else's day with such a note.

"Thanks for the Memories" Retreat

Of all the gifts God gives us in life, are there any we cherish more than fond memories of special occasions with family and friends? I've often thought, "Even if my house burns to the ground and I lose everything, I'll still have my memories." My next thought is usually, "And if I ever smell smoke, I'm grabbing my photo albums first!" Invest in a nice scrapbook, some creative-patterned scissors, and some colorful, acid-free paper and pens. Gather up all those pictures you have tossed into a box over the years and go on this "Thanks for the Memories" retreat with a grateful heart for all the wonderful people in your life and for all the fond moments you've shared. Give thanks to God for each and every photo in your album and pray a special blessing on each face that adorns your pages.

"Leaving a Legacy of Love" Retreat

Take your Bible, pen and paper (or a laptop computer), and plenty of Kleenex tissues for this retreat. The goal is to think back over your life and recall the most spiritually significant moments that shaped who you are. Make a "spiritual time line" from birth to present and map out the spiritual highs and lows of your life. Ask God to show you these spiritual markers and why He caused or allowed these things to happen. Discern how all these things have worked together for your good and for God's glory. Seek to understand what your divine purpose in life has been. Then write a letter to your children explaining these events and communicating how the God who carried you through all of these mountaintops and valleys in life will also be the God who carries them through their brightest and bleakest days. Tell them what you hope they've learned from you and what you want them to remember after you are gone.

My Great-uncle Dorsey (who was also a pastor) did something like this not long before he died. Using a handheld tape recorder and cassette tapes, he told stories from his childhood, memories from his days in World War II, and many of his favorite stories from the pulpit. There are not many family heirlooms treasured more than our own set of Uncle Dorsey's tapes. Taking time to leave behind this unforgettable legacy of love will speak volumes to your children about your faith in Christ and your love for them. It will strengthen their own faith as well.

As you are planning for your special retreat, don't forget to take along a few things to make your time alone with God special and pleasurable to you. Here's a packing list to help you prepare for a memorable retreat:

- intimate worship or powerful Christian contemporary music and a CD player
- an aromatic candle and matches
- bubble bath and a razor to shave your legs
- facial scrub and fragrant body lotion
- manicure kit and nail polish
- duraflame log for a fire in the fireplace if there is one

- your favorite delicacies (leave the peanut butter and jelly at home, Mom! Go for the petite filet mignon and chocolate-covered strawberries!)
- comfy pj's, slippers, and your favorite blanket and pillow
- Bible, a devotional book, a journal, and a pen
- clothes and shoes to walk in

Anticipate this experience as an exciting date. You are running away with your Lover, not confining yourself to a convent. Be creative and bask in the beauty of intimate time alone with God.

However, let me warn you: *Experiencing this incredible pleasure can be very addictive.* My annual retreats have turned into far more frequent excursions. No human can meet our deepest needs like God can, nor should anyone be expected to. My husband doesn't mind granting me this time away because I come back revived, with a renewed sense of joy over being a bride of Christ and a fresh passion for being the wife and mother God has called me to be. I can think of no better way to spend my time.

How about you? Do you need a personal revival and renewed sense of joy? Are you longing for a deeper level of intimacy and fulfillment than a husband can possibly provide? Are you ready to bask in God's special love for you and relish your role as His chosen bride? If so, carve out some special time and a special place to run away and rendezvous with your heavenly Bridegroom.

Your love, O LORD, reaches to the heavens, your faithfulness to the skies. Your righteousness is like the mighty mountains, your justice like the great deep... How priceless is your unfailing love! Both high and low among [women] find refuge in the shadow of your wings. They feast on the abundance of your house; you give them drink from your river of delights.

—*Psalm 36:5-9*

all quiet on the home front

> To [her] who overcomes, I will give the right to sit with me on my
> throne, just as I overcame and sat down with my Father on his throne.
>
> REVELATION 3:21

I recently met a young woman who grew up in the war-torn country of Sierra Leone in West Africa. As bullets whizzed through the city streets and landmines blasted limbs off of children playing in the fields, every day was a struggle for Lela and her family to survive. She had been in the United States less than two years when I asked her what she liked most about living in this country.

She answered with a sweet smile, "Peace. There is nothing like living in peace."

I also asked, "How did you cope with the chaos of war all around you day after day?"

Shrugging her shoulders, she replied, "When war is all you have ever known, you don't realize how chaotic it is."

Although I've never known the terror of dodging bullets or landmines, the truth of Lela's statement struck a chord. I never realized how intense and chaotic my life was until I experienced the peace of living with sexual and emotional integrity. For years I had walked blindly into compromising situations, begged over dinner tables for morsels of affection, and found myself sleeping with the enemy time and time again. I consistently mistook intensity for intimacy and the concept of a peaceful relationship seemed unfathomable.

But God, in His sovereignty, looked beyond my weaknesses and saw my need for genuine intimacy. And in spite of my unfaithfulness, He's been faithful to guide me toward that place of quiet rest in my relationships with my father, my husband,

and myself. This was not an overnight trip from chaos to peacefulness like it was for Lela, but a long process—one that continues to this day.

But before I tell you more about what God has done in me, I want to revisit a couple of the women whose stories were told in the first chapter of this book. They too have moved from the chaotic struggle of sexual compromise to a quiet place of rest.

NO MORE STRANGERS IN THE BEDROOM

Remember Rebecca, who fantasized about being seduced by a stranger in some exotic place in order to have an orgasm while making love with her husband? She now reports:

> I didn't think that what I was doing was wrong at the time. I realize now that Craig was just as hurt over what I was thinking in my mind while we were having sex as I would have been if he had wanted to look at pornography while making love to me. Understanding how we each struggle to maintain sexual integrity has transformed our marriage, our bedroom in particular....
>
> I did what you recommended.... We leave on a dim light and I open my eyes anytime I sense my mind wandering outside of our bedroom. It takes concentration, but when I relax and focus completely on Craig during sex and what we are experiencing together, I feel so close to him and so much closer to God as a result! I actually enjoy sex now rather than just tolerate it and let my mind wander. I never knew it could be this deeply gratifying.
>
> Inappropriate thoughts still try to creep in occasionally, but when I compare our old sex life to this new level of intimacy we've discovered by keeping our minds pure for each other, I'm inspired to redirect my thoughts back to the gift that God gave me in Craig.

Rebecca is right. You will be tempted to resort to your old fantasies, your old masturbation habit, or your dysfunctional relational patterns. That doesn't mean that you can't have victory time and time again, however. With each thought taken captive, each inappropriate word not spoken, each extramarital advance you spurn, and each intimate sexual experience you enjoy with your husband, you will be reinforcing your victory and embracing God's plan for your sexual and emotional fulfillment.

FREE FROM THE WEB OF INTRIGUE

Six years after MiamiMike escorted Jean into his condo for a dip in his hot tub and a sip of champagne, Jean gives this update:

> I wish I could say that I did the right thing that night. I didn't. I lived that whole weekend just like a scene in a movie, but the ending wasn't near as happily ever after as most movies I've watched. After the weekend was over, Mike and I parted ways. He knew I felt guilty and respected my desire for him not to contact me again. I know I was lucky—I've heard horror stories of women being stalked by men that they met over the Internet.
>
> I didn't tell my husband for almost three years, but I felt like the secret was going to rot my insides if I didn't spill it. I never made it through a single day without beating myself up over it, and I had to pretend to enjoy sex with Kevin. All I could think about was, *Would he still love me if he knew my secret?* I felt like I was acting in a play, even with my kids. My secret was keeping me from feeling real at all.
>
> Finally I took Kevin on a weekend vacation without the kids so I could clear my conscience. I told him on the way to the hotel, offering to get separate rooms if he needed some time away from me to think about what he wanted to do. I would have understood completely if he had decided to divorce me. But his response was nothing like I had expected. He said, "Jean, why did you do it?" I explained in tears that I had no good reason to do what I did and that I had regretted that monumental mistake since that weekend.
>
> Then he asked, "Knowing that you could get away with it, why have you never done it again since then?" That question caught me off guard.
>
> "Because that's *not* who I am, Kevin!" I cried, confused and somewhat offended.
>
> "I already knew that, Jean. I just wanted to make sure you know it, too!"

Kevin said compassionately as he wrapped his arms around me and cried, "I'm glad you are still here. I'm glad I didn't lose you forever. We'll get through this."

Kevin's forgiveness wasn't immediate. That took time and several months of marital counseling. But his love and commitment never wavered. I won't say that I am glad I did what I did, but I will say that through this trial our marriage has become more intimate, our communication more open and honest, and we've grown stronger as individuals and as a couple.

We moved our computer to our living room and made a pact with each other not to surf the Internet or go into chat rooms without another person in the room. Kevin says this pact isn't just to keep me safe, but also to keep him from the temptation of looking at Internet pornography. Since all this came out in the open, we are much more honest with each other about our own sexual struggles and emotional temptations, but we have grace for each other and feel a connection that was missing when we kept secrets from each other.

Every time Jean connects with her husband instead of a cyber-buddy, she strengthens her own resolve to avoid compromise at all costs. Although we may have fallen once or even several times, Jean's story reminds us that genuine intimacy and fulfillment are still within our grasp. As you learn who you are in Christ (from the closing exercise of chapter 4), you'll come to understand that you are not a victim of this battle, but a victor! The prize? Peace in your spirit, freedom from disquieting and oppressive thoughts and emotions, harmony in your relationships with God and men, and the sexual fulfillment God longs for you to experience.

MY PAINFUL PAIN-RELIEVING PROCESS

My journey toward the peacefulness of sexual integrity began in 1996 with several months of individual and group counseling. There, by ripping up phone books and screaming at empty chairs instead of at the innocent people I lived with at home, I vented my anger toward every person who had ever hurt me. I sat in a chair across from an imaginary "Shannon at fifteen" (the young girl I once was who was about to make all the sexual mistakes that I had just lived through). With my counselor's guidance, I was able to voice my new understanding of the pain and loneliness this fifteen-year-old had felt, sympathize with her naiveté and confusion about her sexual and emotional desires, and forgive her for the bad choices she was making and the pain that her poor judgment would cause me and many others. I wrote letters of forgiveness to my father and mother, one painfully honest set that would never be mailed and another more socially acceptable set that was mailed and received with sincere appreciation. I also wrote a letter of forgiveness to myself. As I looked over my list of previous partners, I recognized that I was looking for love, approval, and acceptance from every authority figure in my life except from my real father and my heavenly Father. I embarked on a mission to get to know both of them better, frequently carving time out for family camping trips and retreats with the Lord.

During this season of growth and healing, I crucified my fleshly desires and buried many bitter memories. My counselor finally kicked me out of her office saying, "You're healed! Go! You don't need me any more!"

Not long after that I sensed God calling me to speak on sexual purity to youth groups, teaching them all the things I wish I had learned when I was their age. But I argued, "Lord, you've got the wrong person! I'm not a trained speaker and my life is certainly no example for young people to follow!" However, through studying the life of Moses in Henry Blackaby's *Experiencing God* workbook, God convinced me that He knew what He was doing and that I was being ridiculous to argue with Him as if He didn't.

My fervency for sexual purity grew until it became a fire in my bones that felt as if it would consume me if I didn't open my mouth and spit out the words. But in hindsight, I see that I fell more in love with speaking than with the Lord. I was still worshiping another god. Pridefully, I assumed that this "dying" deal was a one-time shot, and I thought I had won that battle once and for all. I figured once you are dead, you are dead, right? You can't get "deader"! But I soon discovered that dying to my worldly desires was a daily requirement. My living sacrifice had been crawling off the altar without my awareness.

I continued indulging in "little" temptations here and there, especially in a particular relationship with a friend (I'll call him John). Over the course of many years, John and I occasionally had lunch together and discussed ministry visions and dreams. Our conversations stimulated me mentally and spiritually, and we would often talk at length on the phone, usually while my husband was at work. I thought nothing of it because we weren't hiding anything from anyone.

Over the years we often bantered cute remarks back and forth, but at one point I told my husband that some of John's comments seemed to border on flirtatiousness. Knowing John well himself, Greg dismissed my concern as an overreaction.

However, John's flirting became so obvious that I felt I had to confront him over lunch one day. In response to one of his wisecracks, I said, "It's beginning to sound like you are not just playing around anymore and you are scaring me. I'm a little concerned about our friendship and wonder if we need to establish some firmer boundaries?"

John confirmed my suspicion when he responded, "Why? Are you tempted too?" He went on to say that he had been in love with me for a long time and that he would give up his marriage and ministry if I would run away with him.

Was I tempted? Certainly.

"But how could you have been tempted if you were happily married?" you might ask. Because I had been sowing the seeds of compromise in most of the ways I've warned against in this book. I had compared my husband to John over and over in my mind. I had entertained fantasies of further, more intimate conversations with John. Had I exercised firmer mental, emotional, spiritual, and physical boundaries, John never would have felt the freedom to say the things he did, nor would I have felt so drawn to him emotionally. In hindsight, I can see how I carelessly raced through the green-light levels of attention and attraction, zoomed through to the yellow-light level of affection, right into the red-light level of emotional arousal and attachment by engaging in an emotional affair.

While it would have been easy to place the blame on John, I knew in my heart that I couldn't. You teach people how to treat you, and I had gradually taught John that he could be overly friendly, perhaps even forward with me, and get away with it. The private car rides, occasional lunches, discussing of intimate details of our marriages and ministries, and bantering back and forth with sly jokes and romantic innuendos had paved the way. I'm just thankful that God provided a detour, just as He promised to in 1 Corinthians 10:13: "No temptation has seized you except what is common to [woman]. And God is faithful; he will not let you be tempted beyond what you can bear. *But when you are tempted, he will also provide a way out so that you can stand up under it*" (emphasis added).

God's way out way for me came in the form of an actual detour. Desperate for direction, I accepted a female mentor's invitation to run away for a sabbatical to seek God's will for this increasingly awkward situation. As we were driving, we accidentally missed the exit and continued driving an hour farther down the interstate before we realized we had gone too far. We stopped to ask directions and have lunch in Lindale, Texas. As my friend blessed our burritos, I clearly heard God say to my heart, "Move here."

It seemed that my faith was being put to the test. Could I trust that this direction was truly from God, or was my mind playing tricks on me? Could I practice what I was preaching about remaining sexually pure, or would I indulge in living a double life? Could I leave John without looking back, or had he become an idol that I would cling to? Did I want to resist extramarital temptation enough to give up my ministry, sell my dream house, leave my extended family and friends, and move to a place where nothing was familiar to me? Or did I want to hold on to my own kingdom and stay in my comfort zone? These and tons of other questions whirled around in my mind, but they all boiled down to these: Who did I love more? Who did I trust more? Who would I follow? God or John?

As Greg and I prayed and asked for confirmation that this direction was, in fact, from God, we felt drawn to the story of Abram. In Genesis 12:1, the Lord said to Abram, "Leave your country, your people and your father's household and go to the land I will show you." We decided that we would trust and obey, even though the pathway out of this mess was not clear.

We posted a FOR SALE BY OWNER sign in the yard of our Dallas dream house. It sold in six days, and we had to be out within three weeks. We told a real estate agent we had to find a house in Lindale—and quickly! The first place he led us to had just been put on the market two days prior—a huge, secluded plot of land with an old log cabin home overlooking a creek in the piney woods of East Texas.

While I loved our house in Dallas, this cabin is truly a writer's paradise and a place where God's presence is evident. It is also a stone's throw from the Teen Mania Ministries campus, where God gave me the awesome privilege of giving birth to Well Women Ministries, which helps young women entrenched in sexual and emotional battles. To someone who knew the taste of defeat all too well, the thrill of victory is truly something to be savored—and shared with others.

In Matthew 19:29, Jesus tells his disciples, "Everyone who has left houses or brothers or sisters or father or mother or children or fields for my sake will receive a hundred times as much and will inherit eternal life." True to His word, God has repaid even more than a hundred times everything He asked us to give up for the sake of righteousness. We sacrificed a nice house on a quarter-acre lot in the hustle and bustle of Dallas for a 122-acre plot of land in the quiet countryside. I sacrificed a speaking ministry that reached maybe two hundred youth each year, and now through Teen Mania and other local ministries God allows me to teach over two hundred women each week. But as nice as the increased physical and spiritual territory is, I am often reminded of God's words to Abram: "I am your shield, your very great reward" (Genesis 15:1).

My joy isn't this land or a ministry or even restored self-esteem. My very great reward is all of the intimacies and ecstasies that I experience with the Lord Himself, a relationship that fills me to overflowing, gives me unspeakable joy, and causes all other relationships to pale in comparison.

I'm not promising that God will give you the same physical rewards I received. However, I can promise that He longs to enjoy this kind of intimate relationship with *you*. He also has rewards custom-tailored just for you that will delight your heart the way He has delighted mine. He promises in Matthew 6:33 that, if we seek first His kingdom and His righteousness, His blessings will be added to us as well.

I'm also not promising that God will heal you the same way that He healed me. Healing comes gradually for most women, but God knows the process that will work best for you. He alone knows how to deliver you out of the chaos of compromise into a place of victory.

While I hope you use this book and its accompanying workbook[1] to guide you to a place of mental, emotional, spiritual, and physical integrity, I encourage you all the more to look directly to God to guide you there. He knows the way. Simply rendezvous with Him regularly for direction.

As you seek genuine intimacy with the God who loves you and holds the plan for your sexual and emotional fulfillment, I pray that you not only discover the thrill of victory in this battle, but that you also experience indescribable joy in the journey.

May the God of hope fill you with all joy and peace as you trust in him, so that you may overflow with hope by the power of the Holy Spirit.

Romans 15:13

The battle for emotional and sexual fulfillment is not an easy one because life is full of disappointments. For some women, every day is an invitation to live in a fantasy world that has no match in reality. So if you are married, you must live each day purposefully focused on building a bond with your husband that grows stronger over time, even through tough seasons. The reality of life is that marriage is not easy, and it requires great effort to craft the institution into the awesome union of love that God intended. Though challenging, the rewards of rich intimacy and deep connection are worth the effort.

If you are single—whether never married, divorced, or widowed—you have a different assignment. You must build a stronger, more intimate bond with God. This bond can produce such fulfillment and connection that you will never feel that you are incomplete as a single person. God's plan for you is as rich and abundant as His plan for married women.

But what if you are married to someone who does not want to change or is so damaged he can't change? I wish that somehow we were protected from making poor marriage choices, but we are not. Perhaps you have read this entire book, shaking your head and in tears because you believe that you will never know the depths of intimacy and connection that others experience with their husbands. You may have asked, "What of me? What of a woman who is full of love and desire, trapped in a marriage with something much less of a prince and much more of a beast?"

If you are in such a marriage, I am so sorry. Every time I receive an e-mail from someone like you, I feel great compassion. It must be very difficult for you to get up and get on with your life each day. I know it only deepens the pain that you had a choice of whom to marry and this is the man you chose. Perhaps you were young, naive, or deeply broken when you married. Now you are older, wiser, and healthier yet still living with the consequence of a choice you wish you had never made. Rather than being a book of hope for you, this book may have caused you to feel even more discouraged and disappointed than when you started it. If so, I have some hope for you.

If you are living with a man who is physically, emotionally, sexually, or spiritually abusive, there are some things you need to do to ensure that he experiences the consequences of his behavior. If you have been told to sit and patiently endure your husband's abuse, you have been told wrong. Sitting and doing nothing only enables your husband to continue to be a man that most likely even he despises. If you are in physical danger, leave. If you are so desperate that you feel you cannot leave, then start looking for alternatives now. Find resources that can help you out of your desperation so that you and your children will not be in danger.

If you are not in physical danger, take some steps to see if the relationship can be changed. This will require courage and perseverance. It will also require the help of others. You simply cannot do this alone.

First of all, get some wise counsel. If possible, see a Christian counselor, a trained professional who has a solid reputation. This person can help you as you struggle to stop doing what you have been doing and risk taking some actions that could initiate change. If a professional is not available, find a wise woman in your church or in a recovery group that will walk through this with you. Someone who has been through this can guide you and encourage you.

Second, seek help from other women. One of the reasons you may have entered an unhealthy relationship with a man is the lack of healthy relationships with women. The care and nurture of other women can help you heal. The presence of strong women who love you and support you will help you feel less desperate. With the help of these women, you can discover new solutions and alternatives that you alone would not be able to develop.

Third, create a life for yourself. You have a choice about how you will live. You don't have to live as if you are trapped in someone else's life. Think of activities you could be doing other than feeling sorry for yourself or living in isolation. There may be groups you could join just for fun. Whether it is learning to dance, playing cards, or developing a new skill, there are unexplored opportunities for you to experience with women who care about you. This may not be the life you always hoped for, but it can be a life far more meaningful than you ever imagined.

Over the years I have watched many women make dramatic changes that led to a very satisfying life, even though they had an unsatisfying marriage. Sometimes—but not always—the husband changes as a result. The stronger she becomes and the more diverse her interests and wider her connections, the more he is drawn to her. Initially he may try to squash her efforts at self-expression and development. He may exert more control and be more insulting and abusive. But then this gives way to a greater desire for his wife. But even in cases where this doesn't happen, these women have chosen to live—to have healthy and nurturing relationships with other women and to grow and learn. So reach out and find the friends you need to live the life you want.

If you are to find the life God wants for you, you must do one more thing—you must forgive. This may be the last thing you want to do, but it may be the very thing you need to do most. Your husband may never ask for your forgiveness. Or at times he may say he is sorry only to repeat the offense in a short time. He may be the worst of the worst, but no matter how "bad" he is, you need to find a way to forgive him. Not for his sake, but for yours.

The longer you refuse to forgive him, the longer he has control of you. You may think he doesn't "deserve" forgiveness, but you deserve living beyond the bitterness and resentment that hurts only you. You deserve the freedom that will only come when you let go of all you have against him. This is not an easy or instant process. You may have been so badly hurt that it would take years to forgive him totally. If that is the case, all the more reason to begin the process now.

Many men do not even know the depths of hurt and pain we have caused the women we love. We have a way of rushing through our lives and stumbling over the most important people in them. Please forgive us for the hurt we have caused. Please forgive your husband so you can unshackle yourself from a past you cannot change and destructive feelings you cannot afford to harbor. Forgive the unforgivable and move into the life that is waiting for you.

May God be with you as you courageously go forward and discover a life that has meaning and purpose. I hope and pray that you will be able to experience it with a husband who loves you, but more than that, I hope you learn to live life to its fullest, healthy husband or not.

P.S. If you have found hope, encouragement, or insight from this book, please share your discoveries with your friends or Sunday-school class. You might even consider leading a class or discussion group using the *Every Woman's Battle Workbook*. If you do, please let me know how it goes at sarterburn@newlife.com.

workbook

questions you may have about this workbook

What will the Every Woman's Battle Workbook do for me?

So often women read books and think of all the other people who need to hear its message. However, *Every Woman's Battle* is intended for every woman…especially you. This workbook will help you recognize your own unique struggle with sexual and emotional integrity and how God's plan for your fulfillment may differ from your own less effective plan.

You'll discover ways to guard not only your body, but also your mind, heart, and mouth against sexual compromise. Through thought-provoking questions and soul-searching exercises, you'll begin to see a new sexual revolution taking shape not just in the world, but inside of you.

Is this workbook enough, or do I also need the book *Every Woman's Battle*?

Although you will find excerpts throughout each chapter from the *Every Woman's Battle* book (each one marked at the beginning and end by this symbol: 📖), we recommend that you read along in the book to see the big picture and get the full effect of the concepts presented.

How much time is required? Do I need to work through every part of each chapter?

According to Annette, Dee, Jenny, Karen, and Lori (our gracious "guinea pigs" with this workbook), you should be able to finish each workbook chapter within twenty-five to thirty minutes. While it's important to work through all the questions in each chapter, you may want to spend more time on areas that target your specific needs.

Each chapter contains four parts: Planting Good Seeds (Personally Seeking God's Truth), Weeding Out Deception (Recognizing the Truth), Harvesting Fulfillment (Applying the Truth), and Growing Together (Sharing the Truth in Small-Group Discussion). The first three sections are intended for individual study. They will help you hide God's Word in your heart, recognize and remove things in your heart that hinder you in this battle, and reap the rewards of living a life of sexual and emotional integrity. The last section of each chapter is designed especially for group discussion, although it can also be done individually.

How do I organize a study group?

You'll be amazed at how much more you'll get out of this book and workbook if you go through it with a group of like-minded women. If you don't know of an existing group, start one of your own! Whether it's a Sunday-school class, a group of coworkers, neighbors, or friends, invite some women to review the book and workbook. Most will recognize that there is always room for improvement in the area of sexual and emotional integrity, and the book is designed to have something for every woman regardless of age, marital status, or previous sexual experience.

The time commitment for going through the book and workbook isn't significant. Most women can find an hour each week to read a chapter in the book and answer the corresponding questions in the workbook. In addition, your group will need to meet together twelve times to discuss each chapter, one at a time. Your meetings should be kept to a reasonable amount of time (I recommend sixty to ninety minutes) so everyone will consider it a blessing rather than a burden. If evenings are not a possibility, consider a weekly breakfast or brown-bag lunch meeting.

When women gather to discuss such an intimate topic, the temptation to rabbit-trail with a variety of other "safer" topics can be overwhelming, especially for someone who is uncomfortable at first. Therefore, one person should be designated as the group facilitator to ensure that the conversation stays on track. This facilitator has no responsibilities to teach, lecture, or prepare anything in advance, but simply to begin and end the meeting at the designated times and to make sure the conversation is moving along in a productive manner.

Before you begin meeting, consider allowing people time to invite friends of their own who may want to be a part of such a group. There is nothing more healing than several women coming together, removing masks they may have been hiding behind for years, and getting real with each other about the sexual and emotional issues that are common to all of us. If being so honest with a group of other women evokes feelings of fear and mistrust, I encourage you to turn to Myth 7 in chapter 3 of *Every Woman's Battle*. You are truly not alone in your struggles, and other women need to know that they are not alone, either. Will you be the one to tell them?

You never know, perhaps your group will rescue someone from the pit of inappropriate fantasies, the snare of masturbation, or perhaps you will start a group just before someone you know falls into an emotional or sexual affair. Your accountability group can truly be a lifeline not just for you, but for every woman who participates.

not just a man's battle!

Read chapter 1 in *Every Woman's Battle*.

PLANTING GOOD SEEDS
(Personally Seeking God's Truth)

As you seek to discover God's plan for sexual and emotional fulfillment, these are some good seeds to plant in your heart:

> You have heard that it was said, "Do not commit adultery." But
> I tell you that anyone who looks at a [man longingly] has already
> committed adultery with [him] in [her] heart. (Matthew 5:27-28)

> Among you there must not be even a hint of sexual immorality.
> (Ephesians 5:3)

1. What do these verses say to you?
2. How does your life measure up to these standards?

For hope that you can win the battle for sexual and emotional integrity, a good seed to plant in your heart is 1 Corinthians 10:13:

No temptation has seized you except what is common to [woman]. And God is faithful; he will not let you be tempted beyond what you can bear. But when you are tempted, he will also provide a way out so that you can stand up under it.

3. Rephrase this verse in your own words.

✎ WEEDING OUT DECEPTION
(Recognizing the Truth)

📖 Over the past decade of pursuing my own healing from these (and other) issues, as well as teaching on the topic of sexual purity and restoration, I have come to understand that in some way or another sexual and emotional integrity is a battle that every woman fights.

Many believe that just because they are not involved in a physical, sexual affair they don't have a problem with sexual and emotional integrity. As a result, they engage in thoughts and behaviors that compromise their integrity and rob them of true sexual and emotional fulfillment. 📖

4. Do you agree with the statement that every woman fights the battle for sexual and emotional integrity? Why or why not?
5. Reflect back on the stories in the first chapter. Which one, if any, of these women's stories strikes a chord in you? How has reading her story opened your eyes to your own battle?
6. Circle how often you have engaged in any of the following:

Unhealthy Comparisons	Never	Sometimes	Often	Always
Mental Fantasies	Never	Sometimes	Often	Always
Emotional Affairs	Never	Sometimes	Often	Always
Romance Novels	Never	Sometimes	Often	Always
Soap Operas	Never	Sometimes	Often	Always
Masturbation	Never	Sometimes	Often	Always

Inappropriate Internet Activity	Never	Sometimes	Often	Always
Other Sexual Dysfunction(s)				
_____	Never	Sometimes	Often	Always
_____	Never	Sometimes	Often	Always

7. What areas of compromise do you need to weed out of your life?
8. Specifically, what effect has this activity had on your marriage? on your relationship with God? on your self-esteem?

🪲 HARVESTING FULFILLMENT
(Applying the Truth)

> 📖 I am thrilled to report that our marriage of thirteen years is still going strong and has never been better (although we, like any other couple, still have our moments). I'm thankful I never traded [Greg] in for another model, and even more thankful that he didn't give up on me, either. Together, we have discovered a new level of intimacy that we didn't know existed, all because I stopped comparing and criticizing and began embracing the uniqueness of my spouse. 📖

9. If you were to refrain from any of the compromising activities that you identified and (if you are married) began to focus all of your sexual energies on your husband, what would the result be in your marriage?
10. What would the result be in your relationship with God?
11. What would the result be on your self-esteem?

🍃 GROWING TOGETHER
(Sharing the Truth in Small-Group Discussion)

> 📖 When I hear people say that women don't struggle with sexual issues like men do, I cannot help but wonder what planet they are

from or what rock they have been hiding under. Perhaps what they really mean is, the physical aspect of sexuality isn't an overwhelming temptation for women like it is for men.

Men and women struggle in different ways when it comes to sexual integrity. While a man's battle begins with what he takes in through his eyes, a woman's begins with her heart and her thoughts. A man must guard his eyes to maintain sexual integrity, but because God made women to be emotionally and mentally stimulated, we must closely guard our hearts and minds as well as our bodies if we want to experience God's plan for sexual and emotional fulfillment. A woman's battle is for sexual *and* emotional integrity. 📖

12. Why do you think so many people assume that women do not struggle with sexual issues?

13. What hinders women from recognizing sexual and emotional compromise?

14. Once women recognize it, what hinders us from talking about it with others?

📖 While a man needs mental, emotional, and spiritual connection, his physical needs tend to be in the driver's seat and his other needs ride along in the back. The reverse is true for women. If there is one particular need that drives us, it is certainly our emotional needs. That's why it's said that men *give love to get sex* and women *give sex to get love.* 📖

15. Have you ever given sex in order to get the love you were longing for? If so, did this method work for you? Why or why not?

16. What prompted you to read *Every Woman's Battle* and utilize this workbook?

17. Of the twenty-five questions asked to determine if you were engaged in a battle for sexual and emotional integrity (see pages 15–17), what surprised you? What scared you?

18. What particular question(s) hit home for you, and why?

19. What is the main thing you are hoping to gain over the next twelve weeks from reading *Every Woman's Battle*? working through this workbook? participating in this discussion group?

∞

Lord, thank You that You are a faithful God who provides a way out whenever we are tempted. Thank You for revealing that we are not alone in our struggles for sexual and emotional integrity. As we seek to learn Your truths, weed deception out of our lives, harvest a bumper crop of fulfillment in our relationships, and grow together as sisters in Christ, we ask that You guide our hearts and minds into greater levels of personal holiness. In Jesus' name. Amen.

a new look at sexual integrity

Read chapter 2 in *Every Woman's Battle*.

PLANTING GOOD SEEDS
(Personally Seeking God's Truth)

As you wonder if you can succeed at moving from a place of compromise to a place of sexual and emotional integrity, plant these good seeds in your heart:

> I, the LORD, have called you in righteousness;
>   I will take hold of your hand.
> I will keep you and will make you
>   to be a covenant for the people
>   and a light for the Gentiles,
> to open eyes that are blind,
>   to free captives from prison
>   and to release from the dungeon those
>   who sit in darkness.
>   (Isaiah 42:6-7)

> I can do everything God asks me to with the help of Christ who gives me the strength and power. (Philippians 4:13, TLB)

1. What effect does it have on your confidence level to know that God will hold your hand and lead you from darkness into light? Why?

To remind yourself about the most important things in life and in your relationships, plant the following seed in your heart:

> Love the Lord your God with all your heart and with all your soul and with all your mind. This is the first and greatest commandment. And the second is like it: "Love your neighbor as yourself." All the Law and the Prophets hang on these two commandments. (Matthew 22:37)

2. How well has your life lined up with this verse? What changes do you need to make in order to fulfill these two commandments?

As you think about behaviors you should or should not engage in—including those not specifically forbidden in Scripture—plant this seed in your heart:

> "Everything is permissible"—but not everything is beneficial.
> "Everything is permissible"—but not everything is constructive.
> Nobody should seek [her] own good, but the good of others.
> (1 Corinthians 10:23-24)

3. Rephrase this verse in your own words.

⚘ WEEDING OUT DECEPTION
(Recognizing the Truth)

📖 By definition, our sexuality isn't *what we do*. Even people who are committed to celibacy are sexual beings. Our sexuality is *who we are,* and we were made with a body, mind, heart, and spirit, not just a body. Therefore, sexual integrity is not just about physical chastity. It is about purity in all four aspects of our being (body, mind, heart, and spirit). When all four aspects line up perfectly, our "tabletop" (our life) reflects balance and integrity....

It's no laughing matter when one of the legs of our sexuality buckles, because then our lives can become a slippery slope leading to discontentment, sexual compromise, self-loathing, and emotional brokenness. When this happens, the blessing that God intended to bring richness and pleasure to our lives feels more like a curse that brings great pain and despair. 📖

4. In your dating relationships, where did you believe "the line" of sexual integrity to be? How far was it "okay" to go prior to marriage? Where did this belief come from?

5. If you ever crossed that imaginary line, were you able to back up and reestablish your preexisting standards? Why or why not?

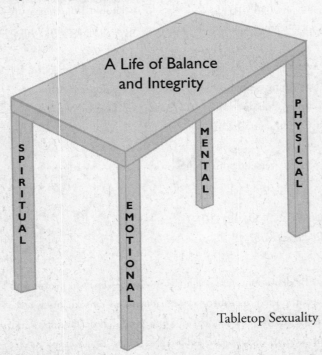

Tabletop Sexuality

6. As you read chapter 2, what insights did you gain about where the line between integrity and compromise should be located?

🦃 Harvesting Fulfillment
(Applying the Truth)

> 📖 In order to have ultimate fulfillment and feel that physical, mental, emotional, and spiritual stability that God intended for us to have, we have to attend to each leg of our table according to God's perfect plan. If one leg is neglected, abused, or attended to in an unrighteous manner, the result is some sort of sexual compromise or emotional brokenness. When each leg is attended to or fulfilled righteously, the result is sexual integrity and emotional wholeness. 📖

7. In what ways are the following needs fulfilled in your life? Are any of these areas in need of attention? If so, how can you attend to these needs in a godly way?

- physical (sexual expression, exercise, proper nutrition)
- mental (educational or professional growth; a balance between stimulation and relaxation)
- emotional (quality time with spouse, family, or friends; enjoying a hobby)
- spiritual (connection with God through prayer, worship, Bible study; ministering to others)

🍃 Growing Together
(Sharing the Truth in Small-Group Discussion)

As someone in the group reads the following passage from *Every Woman's Battle* aloud, one sentence or phrase at a time, underline any phrases that you feel accurately describe you. Put a squiggly line under any phrases that stand out as being things you still need to strive toward.

> 📖 For a Christian woman, sexual and emotional integrity means that her thoughts, words, emotions, and actions all reflect an inner beauty and a sincere love for God, others, and for herself. This doesn't mean she is never tempted to think, say, feel, or do something inappropriate, but she tries diligently to resist these temptations and stands firm in her convictions. She doesn't use men in an attempt to get her emotional cravings met, or entertain sexual or romantic fantasies about men she is not married to. She doesn't compare her husband to other men, discounting his personal worth and withholding a part of herself from him as punishment for his imperfections. She doesn't dress to seek male attention, but she doesn't limit herself to a wardrobe of ankle-length muu-muus, either. She may dress fashionably and look sharp or may even appear sexy (like beauty, sexy is in the eye of the beholder), but her motivation isn't self-seeking or seductive. She presents herself as an attractive woman because she knows she represents God to others.
>
> A woman of integrity lives a life that lines up with her Christian beliefs. She lives according to a standard of love rather than law. She does not claim to be a follower of Christ yet disregard His many teachings on sexual immorality, lustful thoughts, immodest dress, and inappropriate talk. A woman of integrity lives what she believes about God, and it shows everywhere from the boardroom to the bedroom. 📖

8. Share your conclusions (either with the entire group or in smaller groups) about what you see as your strengths and weaknesses when it comes to being a woman of sexual and emotional integrity.

∞

Jesus, thank You for giving us a new look at sexual integrity. Help us to live balanced, healthy lives as we seek to embrace, express, and control our sexuality according to Your perfect plan. In Your precious name we pray. Amen.

seven myths that intensify our struggle

Read chapter 3 in *Every Woman's Battle*.

 PLANTING GOOD SEEDS
(Personally Seeking God's Truth)

As you seek to discern the difference between myth and truth in your battle for sexual and emotional integrity, the following verses hold good seeds to plant in your heart:

> Wisdom is better than weapons of war. (Ecclesiastes 9:18)

1. How can wisdom help you in your battle?

> It is God's will that you should be sanctified: that you should avoid sexual immorality; that each of you should learn to control [her] own body in a way that is holy and honorable, not in passionate lust like the heathen, who do not know God. (1 Thessalonians 4:3-5)

2. Do you believe that God can sanctify you and help you exercise control over your body? Why do you believe what you do? How would your relationships

with men change if you learned to control your body in a way that is holy and honorable?

As you realize your need for God's grace in these matters, plant this in your heart:

> For we do not have a high priest who is unable to sympathize with
> our weaknesses, but we have one who has been tempted in every
> way, just as we are—yet was without sin. Let us then approach the
> throne of grace with confidence, so that we may receive mercy and
> find grace to help us in our time of need. (Hebrews 4:15-16)

3. How does it make you feel to know that Jesus can sympathize with your every weakness (even your sexual weaknesses)? Why?

🔖 WEEDING OUT DECEPTION
(Recognizing the Truth)

> 📖 When we compare ourselves to others, we put one person above
> the other. We either come out on top (producing vanity and pride
> in our lives), or we come up short (producing feelings of disappoint-
> ment with what God gave us). Regardless of how we measure up
> when we make these comparisons, our motives are selfish and sinful
> rather than loving. 📖

4. Have you compared yourself with other women or your husband to other men? In what ways? What has been the result?

> 📖 When you fantasize about someone else when making love with
> your husband, you are mentally making love with another man. *He*,
> not your husband, is the one you feel passionate about. *He*, not
> your husband, is the one you feel close to emotionally. 📖

5. Do you agree or disagree with the above statements? Why or why not?

6. Have you ever fantasized about another man while making love to your husband? How did this affect your ultimate fulfillment?

> 📖 "If sin doesn't know you, it won't call your name!" Once the sin of masturbation does know you by name, it *will* call. And call… and call…and call…. The only way to kill a bad habit is to *starve it to death*. Starving a bad habit can be painful, but not as painful as letting it rule over you. 📖

7. If masturbation has been an issue for you, what benefit have you believed it would bring? What effect has masturbation had on your thought life and on your ability to control your body in relationships with men?

🍂 HARVESTING FULFILLMENT
(Applying the Truth)

> 📖 God gives us grace to accept our husbands and ourselves as we really are, and He gives us the ability to truly love one another unconditionally and unreservedly.
>
> If we crave genuine intimacy, we must learn to seek it only in this kind of grace-filled relationship. The word *intimacy* itself can best be defined by breaking it into syllables: *in-to-me-see*. Can we see into one another and respect, appreciate, and value what is really there, regardless of how that measures up to anyone else? That is what unconditional love and relational intimacy is all about, and this type of intimacy can be discovered only by two people who are seeking sexual and emotional integrity with all their mind, body, heart, and soul. 📖

8. Do you have any reservations about your husband (or those closest to you) seeing into every part of you? Why or why not? What, if anything, do you hide from your husband (or those closest to you)—and why?

9. As intimacy blossoms in your marriage and you see into your husband's heart and mind, how can you give him the same grace that God gives to you? What things about him might you need to accept in order to love him unconditionally and unreservedly?

> 📖 Put all your eggs in one basket. Invest in the relationship you've got. Focus on your marriage wholeheartedly, as if no other man existed. Assume that your spouse is the man you will grow old with. Your husband is God's gift to you. Unwrap the gift and enjoy him for as long as you have him. 📖

10. In order for you to invest all that you've got into your marriage relationship, what needs to change? How will this affect your relationship with your husband? How will this, in turn, affect your level of fulfillment?

❧ Growing Together
(Sharing the Truth in Small-Group Discussion)

> 📖 Sixty-seven percent of all women will experience at least one or more premarital or extramarital affair in her lifetime.[1] That is the number of women who *give in* to these temptations. I believe the percentage is much higher (I'm guessing in the 90 percent range) of those women who simply experience the temptation to engage in premarital or extramarital affairs. 📖

11. Did you find this statistic surprising? Why or why not?
12. Which of the seven myths discussed in chapter 3 are ones that you have previously bought into? How has believing these myths intensified your struggle?

---

1. Tim Clinton, from a class titled "Counselor Professional Identity, Function and Ethics Videotape Course," External Degree Program, Liberty University, Lynchburg, Va. Used with permission.

13. As you read about these myths, did God speak to you about an issue that is currently keeping you from discovering His plan for your sexual and emotional fulfillment? What did you feel God was revealing to you, and why?

14. What are you doing to incorporate this truth into your daily life?

15. Do you have someone you could ask to help hold you accountable in your battle for sexual and emotional integrity? Are you willing to be held accountable in this area? Why or why not?

∞

*F*ather God, thank You for giving us Your truth and dispelling the myths that cloud our judgment. We acknowledge that all wisdom comes from You and that Your truth is all we need to set us free to enjoy healthy relationships. In Your Son's name we pray. Amen.

time for a new revolution

Read chapter 4 in *Every Woman's Battle*.

🪴 PLANTING GOOD SEEDS
(Personally Seeking God's Truth)

As you seek to become the person that God designed you to be, a good seed to plant in your heart is:

> [God] is looking for those with changed hearts and minds. Whoever
> has that kind of change in [her] life will get [her] praise from God.
> (Romans 2:29, TLB)

1. How has your life conformed to worldly patterns? How do your heart and mind need to be changed in order to avoid conforming to such patterns any longer?

As you reclaim God's gift of authority over Satan and the world and exercise self-control, a good seed to plant in your heart is Galatians 5:22-23:

> But the fruit of the Spirit is love, joy, peace, patience, kindness,
> goodness, faithfulness, gentleness and self-control.

2. Which fruit of the Spirit do you feel is evident in your life? Which are in need of further development and why?

3. As you seek to fully understand who God made you to be, some good seeds to plant in your heart are the scriptures listed in the "Who I Am in Christ" chart at the close of chapter 4 (pages 61–63). Which of these scriptures stand out to you as having the power to transform your life if you embraced them and lived accordingly? (Remember that the thirty-day challenge of reciting these scriptures daily will help you internalize who you are in Christ.)

✎ WEEDING OUT DECEPTION
(Recognizing the Truth)

📖 I was seeking to understand why I still felt tempted outside of my marriage, so my therapist asked me to spend a week making a list of every man I had ever been with sexually or had pursued emotionally. I was shocked and saddened to see how long my list had grown through the years.

At the next visit, she asked me to spend a week praying and asking myself, "What do each of these men have in common?" God showed me that each relationship had been with someone who was older than I and in some form of authority over me—my professor, my boss, my lawyer.

As I searched my soul to discern why such a common thread existed in my relational pursuits, the root of the issue became evident: my hunger for power over a man. 📖

4. If you were to create a list of the men you have had sexual experiences with, pursued emotionally (or allowed to pursue you), or fantasized about, what common threads do you think would surface? (If it would help to make a list, do so on a separate sheet of paper that can be destroyed later.)

5. What have you hoped to gain from previous sexual relationships, emotional entanglements, or inappropriate fantasies (power, status, excitement, distraction from boredom or pressure, attention, affirmation, affection, security, and so on)?

6. What do you suspect may be the root issue that has driven you toward such behavior?

7. Do you believe that what you are looking for can truly be found in an unhealthy relationship or in fantasy? If so, have you found it? If not, where would be a better place to look?

🌾 HARVESTING FULFILLMENT
(Applying the Truth)

> 📖 In my attempts to fill the father-shaped hole in my heart and establish some semblance of self-worth through these dysfunctional relationships, I was creating a long list of shameful liaisons and a trunk load of emotional baggage. I was overlooking the only true source of satisfaction and self-worth: an intimate relationship with my heavenly Father. Through pursuing this relationship first and foremost, not only has Jesus become my first love and given me a sense of worth beyond what any man could give, He has also restored my relationship with my earthly father and helped me remain faithful to my husband. 📖

8. Do you believe that you can have an intimate and satisfying relationship with God? Why or why not? What are you currently doing to pursue this kind of relationship with God?

9. What would be the result if every woman on the planet discovered God's plan for sexual and emotional fulfillment and lived accordingly?

10. Do you believe that God truly desires sexual and emotional fulfillment for your life? for every woman's life? Write your response in the form of a prayer,

asking God for this fulfillment for you and for every other woman (or asking for faith to believe it is possible).

🌿 GROWING TOGETHER
(Sharing the Truth in Small-Group Discussion)

11. What is the most beneficial nugget of wisdom that you gleaned from this chapter? Why?

> 📖 Rather than use what beauty God had given me to bring glory to Him, I used it as bait to lure men into feeding my ego. Rather than inspiring men to worship God, I subconsciously wanted them to worship me, and if I was successful in hooking a man with my charms, I felt secretly powerful. 📖

12. What do you feel is the reason that God gives physical assets to a woman (an attractive body, a lovely face, beautiful eyes, a brilliant smile, or a magnetic personality)? What responsibilities come along with these gifts? How should we use these gifts? How should we not use them?

13. Do you use the physical assets that God gave you to glorify *yourself* rather than Him? Explain your answer.

> 📖 Turning the tide in our culture may seem like an impossible task, but we are not alone in this challenge. *God* will turn the tide *through* us. He simply asks us to submit our own lives to Him and to be a witness to what His power and love can do. As more and more women receive this revelation and share this wisdom with others, the tide will eventually turn on its own. We need to begin by focusing on our own behaviors so that we no longer allow the world to influence us. This can only be done by personally reclaiming the gift of authority that Eve originally gave away. 📖

14. If you believe it is time for a new revolution, what specifically can you do in order to:

  • exercise your God-given authority and seek to understand who you are in Christ?
  • embrace God's plan for sexual and emotional fulfillment?
  • keep the world from leading you back into compromise?
  • inspire other women to pursue sexual and emotional integrity?

Heavenly Father, we acknowledge that our society has strayed far from Your plan for sexual and emotional fulfillment. It is truly time for a new sexual revolution, and we pray that it would begin today in each of us. In Jesus' name. Amen.

taking thoughts captive

Read chapter 5 in *Every Woman's Battle.*

🌱 PLANTING GOOD SEEDS
(Personally Seeking God's Truth)

As you recognize that the battle for sexual and emotional integrity begins in the mind, a good seed to plant in your heart is 2 Corinthians 10:3-5:

> For though we live in the world, we do not wage war as the world
> does. The weapons we fight with are not the weapons of the world....
> We take captive every thought to make it obedient to Christ.

1. How is taking thoughts captive a weapon against sexual and emotional compromise? Is it a weapon you've learned to use effectively? Why or why not?

As you are tempted to pursue sexual and emotional fulfillment the world's way, Romans 12:1-2 is a good seed to plant in your heart:

> Therefore, I urge you, [sisters], in view of God's mercy, to offer your
> bodies as living sacrifices, holy and pleasing to God—this is your
> spiritual act of worship. Do not conform any longer to the pattern

of this world, but be transformed by the renewing of your mind.
Then you will be able to test and approve what God's will is—
his good, pleasing and perfect will.

2. Using your own words, describe what Paul was saying in each of his three sentences above.

WEEDING OUT DECEPTION
(Recognizing the Truth)

In the movie *What Women Want,* Nick Marshall (Mel
Gibson) develops a telepathic ability to hear each thought,
opinion, and desire that goes through every woman's head.

Imagine this: Tomorrow morning you wake up and every
man on the planet has developed the ability to read your mind
just by being in your presence. Does the thought make you
nervous?...

Even though we can rest assured that men and women aren't
likely to develop this sensitivity anytime soon, we have an even
bigger concern. God has had this ability all along. Could you,
like David, be so bold as to pray such a thing as this: "Test
me, O LORD, and try me, examine my heart and my mind"
(Psalm 26:2)?

3. How does it make you feel to know that God is fully aware of your each and
every thought? What effect do the inappropriate thoughts we entertain have
on God's heart? Why?

4. Are you, like David, *eager* for the Holy Spirit to examine your mind and test
your thoughts? Why or why not?

Consider the following verse:

> I am jealous for you with a godly jealousy. I promised you to one
> husband, to Christ, so that I might present you as a pure virgin to
> him. But I am afraid that just as Eve was deceived by the serpent's
> cunning, your minds may somehow be led astray from your sincere
> and pure devotion to Christ. (2 Corinthians 11:2-3)

5. How consistent have you been in your devotion to Christ? What things keep your mind from being fully devoted to Him?
6. What specific things can you do to restore your devotion to Christ? What effect will this have on your thought life? on your ability to resist temptation?

🐚 HARVESTING FULFILLMENT
(Applying the Truth)

> Sow a thought, reap an action:
> Sow an action, reap a habit;
> Sow a habit, reap a character;
> Sow a character, reap a destiny.
> —Samuel Smiles

7. What specific things do you feel that God designed you to accomplish in life? What roles do you want to be fondly remembered for at the end of your life?
8. Describe the character traits of such a person who accomplished these things or fulfilled these roles you listed.
9. What regular actions and habits would a person of such character practice?
10. Does your thought life equip you or hinder you from being the person God designed you to be and from fulfilling the destiny that He has for you? How so?
11. What specific recurring thoughts do you need to take captive in order for you to be all that God made you to be? Are you willing to surrender those and make them obedient to Christ?

♣ GROWING TOGETHER
(Sharing the Truth in Small-Group Discussion)

12. What in this chapter was most helpful to you? Why?

13. What new line of defense do you plan to incorporate into your life in order to resist temptation at the gate? redirect tempting thoughts? renew your mind?

14. What does the following saying mean to you? How would you explain it to a younger woman?

> You *can't* keep a bird from flying over your head, but you *can* keep him from building a nest in your hair!

15. How do you keep "birds" from "building a nest in your hair?" In other words, how do you distract yourself in order to avoid entertaining random, inappropriate thoughts?

> 📖 We are rehearsing when we think about the conversations we would have with a particular man if we were ever alone with him, when we entertain thoughts of an intimate rendezvous, or wish that a certain man would take special notice of us.... Then when Satan lays the trap and leads that man in your direction, guess what? We are more than likely going to play the part exactly the way we have rehearsed it. When we don't guard our minds in our relationships with men, we weaken our resistance before any encounter takes place. 📖

16. Do you agree that our thoughts are often rehearsals for how we behave in the face of temptation? Why or why not?

17. Share with the group an example of how you either succumbed to or resisted temptation because of how you rehearsed your part in your thoughts. What did you learn from this experience?

∞

Holy Spirit, search our minds and reveal those thoughts hindering our ultimate fulfillment in relationships with others and with You. Continue to teach us to take every thought captive and make it obedient to Christ. In Jesus' name. Amen.

guarding your heart

Read chapter 6 in *Every Woman's Battle*.

🜊 PLANTING GOOD SEEDS
(Personally Seeking God's Truth)

As you seek to understand the pivotal role that your heart plays in your sexual, emotional, and spiritual life, some good seeds to plant in your heart include:

> Above all else, guard your heart,
>   for it is the wellspring of life.
>   (Proverbs 4:23)

> I the LORD search the heart
>   and examine the mind,
> to reward a [woman] according to [her] conduct,
>   according to what [her] deeds deserve.
>   (Jeremiah 17:10)

1. According to these passages, why should you guard your heart?

As you seek to align your life with God's plan for sexual and emotional fulfillment, a good seed to plant in your heart is:

You know the next commandment pretty well, too: "Don't go to bed with another's spouse." But don't think you've preserved your virtue simply by staying out of bed. Your *heart* can be corrupted by lust even quicker than your *body*. (Matthew 5:27, MSG)

2. What do you think Jesus was saying to His disciples in this passage? What does the passage say to you personally?

🖌 WEEDING OUT DECEPTION
(Recognizing the Truth)

📖 While the need to love and to feel loved is a universal cry of the heart, the problem lies in where we look for this love. If we are not getting the love we need or want from a man—whether or not we have a husband—we may go searching for it. Some look in bars and others in business offices. Some look on college campuses and some look in churches. Some women look to male friends while others look to fantasy. When love eludes them, some women seek to medicate the pain of loneliness or rejection. Some take solace in food; others in sexual relationships with any willing partner. Some turn to soap operas; others to shopping; and still others to self-gratification.

If you have tried any of these avenues for long, you have likely come to a dead end. Your pursuit has left you longing for something greater, something deeper, something more. 📖

3. Have you looked for love in problematic places? If so, where did you look, and what was the result?
4. How have you sought to medicate the pain of loneliness or rejection? How has this worked for you?

📖 Rather than running to the Ultimate Healer for relief from our emotional wounds, women often make idols of relationships—worshiping a man instead of God. We begin submitting to a man's and our own unholy desires rather than submitting to God's desires for our holiness and purity, thus becoming a slave to our passions.

When we peel back the layers of this issue, we can see the core problem: *doubt that God can truly satisfy our innermost needs*. So we look to a man who is not our husband and eventually discover that he doesn't "fix" us, either. 📖

5. Do you believe that at the core of sexual and emotional compromise is *doubt* that God is truly sufficient to satisfy our innermost needs? Why or why not?

6. Do *you* doubt that God can meet *your* deepest needs? If so, write a prayer to God confessing this doubt and asking Him to remove it. If not, write a prayer affirming your belief that He is sufficient.

📖 [God] wants to dwell in every part of your heart, not just rent a room there. He wants to fill your heart to overflowing.

Don't let guilt from past mistakes keep you from seeking this truly satisfying first-love relationship with Him. God does not despise you for the way you've tried to fill the void in your heart. He says, "Come now, let us reason together.... Though your sins are like scarlet, they shall be white as snow; though they are red as crimson, they shall be like wool" (Isaiah 1:18). He is eager to cleanse your heart and teach you how to guard it from future pain and loneliness. 📖

7. Does God dwell in your heart or just rent a room there? Does a guilty heart hinder you from experiencing the fullness of God's unconditional love for you? Why or why not?

🐚 HARVESTING FULFILLMENT
(Applying the Truth)

8. In your own words, explain the stages of the green-light level of emotional connection and why these are acceptable. (Please reference the illustration on the next page.)

   Attraction

   Attention

9. In your own words, explain the stages of the yellow-light level of emotional connection and why we need to exercise caution with these stages.

   Emotional Arousal and Attachment (single women only)

   Affection

10. Finally, explain the stages of the red-light level and why we need to stop before crossing these lines.

    Emotional Affairs and Addictions

    Emotional Arousal and Attachment (married women only)

    📖 As you use caution and strive to refrain from red-light stages of emotional connection, you will regain the self-control, dignity, and self-respect you may have lost if you have compromised your sexual integrity. You can also expect a renewed sense of connection and intimacy with your husband and purity in your friendships or work relationships with other men. But best of all, when God looks on your pure heart and sees that you are guarding it against unhealthy relationships, He will reward you with an even greater revelation of Himself. 📖

11. What gives you the most incentive for avoiding the red-light stages of emotional connection? What specifically can you do to avoid crossing the line between integrity and compromise?

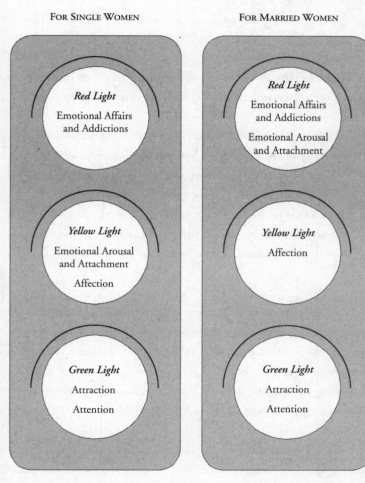

For Single Women	For Married Women
Red Light — Emotional Affairs and Addictions	**Red Light** — Emotional Affairs and Addictions / Emotional Arousal and Attachment
Yellow Light — Emotional Arousal and Attachment / Affection	**Yellow Light** — Affection
Green Light — Attraction / Attention	**Green Light** — Attraction / Attention

Identifying Green, Yellow, and Red Levels of Emotional Connection

❧ GROWING TOGETHER
(Sharing the Truth in Small-Group Discussion)

12. What was the most beneficial thing you learned in chapter 6 about guarding your heart? Why was this helpful to you?

13. How would your life have been different had you learned about guarding your heart before you started dating?

14. If (or when) you have children, how can you share with them the concepts about guarding your heart that would have benefited you as a teenager?

Consider the following passage from *Every Woman's Battle,* then break into smaller groups and answer the questions adapted from the close of chapter 6.

> 📖 While avoiding unhealthy emotional connections and relationships is important, it's not enough to guarantee success in keeping our hearts guarded against compromise. The secret to ultimate emotional satisfaction is to pursue a mad, passionate love relationship with the One who made our hearts, the One who purifies our hearts, and the One who strengthens our hearts against worldly temptations. The secret is to focus your heart on your First Love. 📖

15. Have I *really* invested much time getting to know God personally and intimately? What have I done to get to know God?

16. Have I given God as many chances as I have given other men? fantasy? Internet chat rooms?

17. Am I willing to make the choice to pray or to dance to worship music or to go for a walk with God instead of picking up the phone to call a guy when I am lonely?

18. Am I willing to invite God to satisfy my every need by letting go of all the things, people, and thoughts that I use to medicate my pain, fear, or loneliness so that I might become totally dependent upon Him?

19. After answering these questions, can you honestly say that Jesus Christ is truly your first love? If not, what can you do to enhance the intimacy in your relationship with Him?

∞

Create in me a pure heart, O God, and renew a steadfast spirit within me. Do not cast me from your presence or take your Holy Spirit from me. Restore to me the joy of your salvation and grant me a willing spirit, to sustain me. Then I will teach transgressors your ways, and sinners will turn back to you (prayer of David, Psalm 51:10-13).

locking loose lips

Read chapter 7 in *Every Woman's Battle*.

PLANTING GOOD SEEDS
(Personally Seeking God's Truth)

As you consider the effect of your words on your relationship with God, with others, and with yourself, some good seeds to plant in your heart are:

> If anyone considers [herself] religious and yet does not keep a tight rein on [her] tongue, [she] deceives [herself] and [her] religion is worthless. (James 1:26)

> The tongue is a small part of the body, but it makes great boasts. Consider what a great forest is set on fire by a small spark. The tongue is also a fire, a world of evil among the parts of the body. It corrupts the whole person, sets the whole course of his life on fire. (James 3:5-6)

1. What do these verses say to you?

As you seek to integrate your words with your life of sexual and emotional integrity, plant these seeds in your heart:

> For out of the overflow of the heart the mouth speaks. The good [woman] brings good things out of the good stored up in [her], and the evil [woman] brings evil things out of the evil stored up in [her]. But I tell you that [women] will have to give account on the day of judgment for every careless word they have spoken. For by your words you will be acquitted, and by your words you will be condemned. (Matthew 12:34-37)

> But among you there must not be even a hint of sexual immorality, or of any kind of impurity…because these are improper for God's holy people. Nor should there be obscenity, foolish talk or course joking which are out of place, but rather thanksgiving. (Ephesians 5:3-4)

2. Do you agree that the words that flow from your mouth are actually a reflection of what is in your heart? Why or why not?

⚘ WEEDING OUT DECEPTION
(Recognizing the Truth)

> 📖 What is a four-letter word for a woman's favorite foreplay activity? T-A-L-K!
>   Think about it. What affair has ever taken place without intimate words exchanged? Women often tell me, "I've not been unfaithful to my husband. All this man and I have done is talk." 📖

3. Do you feel that a man or woman can be unfaithful simply because of the words they exchange with a person other than his or her spouse? Why or why not?

📖 While it may be okay to act amorously (as if desiring romance) toward someone you are interested in developing a mutually benefi- cial relationship with, flirting is a different matter. Flirting could also be called "teasing," as the person doing the flirting has no serious intent. 📖

4. Do you think it is okay for a woman—even a single woman—to flirt with a man if she has no intention of investing in a romantic relationship? Explain.
5. If you enjoy flirting with men, what do you think you might be looking to gain? Has flirting ever put you in an uncomfortable or compromising situa- tion? Explain your answer.

📖 Women can be far too nurturing in situations, even when red flags begin to surface. We often think, *But he needs me... I'm just trying to be a friend... How can I possibly* not *help? That would not be very Christianlike!* 📖

6. Do you tend to be overly nurturing with men, frequently playing the "mother" or "counselor" or "best friend" role? If so, what may be behind this tendency?
7. Have you experienced temptations to compromise your sexual and emotional integrity because you were being "too good for your own good?" If so, how can you overcome this tendency?

🦬 HARVESTING FULFILLMENT
(Applying the Truth)

📖 If we long to be women of sexual and emotional integrity, we must understand what a mighty weapon our words are. Words are what will lead us into an affair, or words will stop an affair before it ever begins. 📖

8. Do you agree that a woman can either start or avoid an affair simply by the words she allows to come out of her mouth? Why or why not?

9. Suppose a friend tells you, "I don't want to fall into an affair, but I feel I must be honest with this man about my feelings for him." How would you respond? Does being a woman of integrity mean that we must always be open and honest about our feelings with the object of our temptation? Why or why not?

10. Let's suppose that you have feelings for a particular man, but you refuse to act on them or confess them to anyone other than God and an accountability partner. How do you think that would make you feel to display such strength in the face of temptation? How might you benefit from this choice spiritually and emotionally?

📖 In our quest for relational intimacy, remember that there is Someone we can whisper our heart's desires to and get our boosts from who isn't going to jeopardize our integrity but will strengthen it.

If you are thinking, *No way will talking to God ever excite me like talking to a man will,* then you haven't allowed yourself to be courted by our Creator. The same God whose words possessed the power to form the entire universe longs to whisper words into your hungry heart that have the power to thrill you, heal you, and draw you into a deeper love relationship than you ever imagined possible. A guy may say that you look fine, but God's Word says, "The king is enthralled by your beauty" (Psalm 45:11). A man may tell you, "Of course I love you," but God says, "I have loved you with an everlasting love; I have drawn you with loving-kindness" (Jeremiah 31:3). Even your husband may tell you, "I'm committed to you until death," but God says, "Never will I leave you; never will I forsake you." (Hebrews 13:5) 📖

11. If you have experienced such affirmations from God, how can they sustain you in times of emotional longing outside of marriage? Or if you have never

experienced such intimacy and ecstasy in your relationship with God, how might you cultivate that?

♣ GROWING TOGETHER
(Sharing the Truth in Small-Group Discussion)

12. What were the most valuable lessons you took from this chapter? How can you hold on to them and draw from them in times of temptation?

> 📖 It has been said that men use conversation as a means of communicating information, but women use conversation as a means of bonding. While communicating and bonding with our spouses, children, or female friends is great, communicating and bonding with men outside our marriage or with men we wouldn't choose to date is dangerous and often destructive. And yes, the more we communicate with a person, the more we bond, so we would do well to take a lesson from the men in this area and learn to stick to business a little better. We can learn to communicate with men in friendly but to-the-point ways that will not jeopardize our emotional integrity. 📖

13. Have you ever bonded with a man unintentionally due to excess communication? What did you learn from this experience?
14. What boundaries have you implemented (or may need to implement) to keep from bonding with men in inappropriate ways, whether in person, over the phone, or in cyberspace?
15. If you never exchange inappropriate words with a man (in person, over the phone, or in cyberspace), what is the likelihood that you will fall into a sexual affair?
16. How does it make you feel to know that resisting an emotional or sexual affair may be as easy as choosing appropriate words and avoiding inappropriate words? Is this revelation a relief to you? Why or why not?

∞

Lord, impress upon us the magnitude of the power that our words possess. We ask You to sanctify our speech at all times and with all people. Teach us to use our words to draw attention to You rather than to ourselves. Help us to speak blessings into other people's lives and to listen carefully as You speak blessings over us. In Jesus' name. Amen.

building better boundaries

Read chapter 8 in *Every Woman's Battle*.

PLANTING GOOD SEEDS
(Personally Seeking God's Truth)

As you seek to evaluate what weak links may exist in your armor of protection against sexual and emotional compromise, a good seed to plant in your heart is 1 Corinthians 6:19-20:

> Do you not know that your body is a temple of the Holy Spirit, who is in you, whom you have received from God? You are not your own; you were bought at a price. Therefore honor God with your body.

1. What did Paul mean when he said our bodies are a "temple of the Holy Spirit"? How might this concept change a woman's view of her sexual conduct? How can we honor God with our bodies?

As you consider whether your personal boundaries may need to be strengthened, plant Galatians 6:7-8 in your heart:

> Do not be deceived: God cannot be mocked. A [woman] reaps what [she] sows. The one who sows to please [her] sinful nature, from that nature will reap destruction; the one who sows to please the Spirit, from the Spirit will reap eternal life.

2. Based on the sexual or relational seeds you are currently sowing, what can you
   expect to reap? Explain your answer.

As you seek to believe that your ultimate value comes from your attitude toward
God rather than your appearance, some good seeds to plant in your heart are these:

> I also want women to dress modestly, with decency and propriety,
> not with braided hair or gold or pearls or expensive clothes, but
> with good deeds, appropriate for women who profess to worship
> God. (1 Timothy 2:9-10)

> Charm is deceptive, and beauty is fleeting;
> > but a woman who fears the LORD is to be praised.
> Give her the reward she has earned,
> > and let her works bring her praise at the city gate.
> > > (Proverbs 31:30-31)

3. What do you think it means to fear the Lord? How might a woman benefit
   from becoming a woman who fears the Lord?
4. Why do you think women often fear other people's opinion of their appearance more than they fear God's opinion of their hearts? Which of these
   describes you? How do you think a woman can change her focus from being
   concerned about how she looks to being more concerned with the condition
   of her heart?

WEEDING OUT DECEPTION
(Recognizing the Truth)

> 📖 While the Bible doesn't specifically state how long a skirt should
> be or what sections of skin should always be covered, we can always
> go back to Jesus' commandment as a guideline for how we are to
> dress: Love your neighbor as yourself. 📖

5. Are you prone to dress for attention rather than to dress for respect? Why or why not?

6. Close your eyes and imagine standing in front of your closet. What clothes do you have that are likely to tempt a man to lust after your body? Are you willing to sacrifice the ego boost you may get from wearing those clothes for the sake of loving your neighbor?

> 📖 The only way to truly protect yourself is to guard against sexual compromise altogether. No condom fully protects you against the physical consequences of sexually immoral behavior. Even more important, no condom protects you against the spiritual consequences of sin (broken fellowship with God). No condom will protect you from the emotional consequences of a broken heart. Therefore, don't think in terms of "safe sex," but in terms of "saving sex" until marriage or remarriage. Wise is the woman who avoids compromising behavior that can put her body at risk of disease. 📖

7. Have you jeopardized your sexual integrity because you believed that using a condom during intercourse constitutes "safe sex"? Why do some people make the assumption that as long as a woman doesn't get pregnant or contract a disease that sex outside of marriage is okay?

8. Even if a woman escapes the physical consequences of premarital sex, what emotional and spiritual consequences may she face?

🦫 HARVESTING FULFILLMENT
(Applying the Truth)

> 📖 You have probably heard gourmet chefs on the cooking channel say that when it comes to food, presentation is everything. Presentation *is* everything, not just with food, but also with your body. One of the concepts that I impress upon women is that we teach people

how to treat us. We either teach them to treat us with respect or we teach them to treat us with disrespect. 📖

9. Do you agree that the way a woman dresses affects whether others treat her with respect or disrespect? Explain your answer.

10. Has reading *Every Woman's Battle* raised any convictions within you about changing the way you present yourself with a certain person or in a certain setting? Explain your answer.

> 📖 When you spend time with someone, you are giving that person a gift: *your presence.* It's true. The gift of your company is very precious and of value beyond description. Underneath your breasts lies a beating heart where the Holy Spirit makes His home. Behind your face is a brain that possesses the mind of Christ. Be wary of men who are intrigued by the wrapping but fail to see the value of what is inside the package. They may want to play with the bow...untie the ribbon...peek through the wrapping. 📖

11. Do you consider your presence a gift to those with whom you choose to spend your time? Why or why not?

12. If you felt that you were appreciated more for your heart, mind, and spirit than for your "outer wrapping," how might it change how you feel about yourself?

13. How can you strengthen your emphasis on the "inner package" so that your beauty radiates from within?

❧ GROWING TOGETHER
(Sharing the Truth in Small-Group Discussion)

> 📖 Your body is the temple of the Holy Spirit; your heart, God's dwelling place. As a believer, you have the mind of Christ. And your words are instruments of His wisdom and encouragement to others.

When you put on the full armor of God and vigilantly guard your
body, heart, mind, and mouth without compromise, you are well
on your way to reaping the physical, emotional, mental, and spiritual benefits of sexual integrity. 📖

14. Do you wholeheartedly believe that your body is a temple of the Holy Spirit?
that your heart is God's dwelling place? that you have the mind of Christ?
that your words are God's instrument of wisdom and encouragement to
others? Why or why not?

15. If you were to embrace these truths, believing each of them to be your
birthright as a believer in Christ, what effect would it have on your self-
esteem? on your relationships?

16. As a result of reading the past four chapters in the part of *Every Woman's Battle*
titled "Designing a New Defense," what new ways have you learned to guard
your body, heart, mind, and mouth against compromise?

17. What do you believe the physical, emotional, mental, and spiritual benefits of
sexual integrity to be? What benefits are you already enjoying? What benefits
do you hope to gain?

∞

*Father God, where would we be were it not for Your divine
protection? Thank you for teaching us appropriate physical and
relational boundaries so that we may guard the temple of Your
Holy Spirit. Continue to instill in each of us a sense of modesty
and propriety so that we can reflect Your glorious image to all
we encounter. In Jesus' holy and precious name. Amen.*

sweet surrender

Read chapter 9 in *Every Woman's Battle*.

PLANTING GOOD SEEDS
(Personally Seeking God's Truth)

As you let go of past emotional pain and seek to reconcile relationships, a good seed to plant in your heart is James 3:17-18:

> But the wisdom that comes from heaven is first of all pure; then peace-loving, considerate, submissive, full of mercy and good fruit, impartial and sincere. Peacemakers who sow in peace raise a harvest of righteousness.

1. What do you think it means to "sow in peace"? How does an unwillingness to forgive affect one's life? marriage? fulfillment?

As you surrender your pride, embrace humility, and recognize that nothing short of God's grace will help you overcome sexual temptations, a good seed to plant in your heart is Titus 2:11:

> For the grace of God that brings salvation has appeared to all [women]. It teaches us to say "No" to ungodliness and worldly

passions, and to live self-controlled, upright and godly lives in
this present age, while we wait for the blessed hope—the glorious
appearing of our great God and Savior, Jesus Christ, who gave
himself for us to redeem us from all wickedness and to purify for
himself a people that are his very own, eager to do what is good.

2. Do you believe that God's grace to resist sexual sin is available to anyone who
believes in Christ? Why or why not?

3. Are you eager to live a self-controlled, upright, and godly life? Do you feel
that God's grace is sufficient for you to live such a life? Why or why not?

WEEDING OUT DECEPTION
(Recognizing the Truth)

📖 If you want to win the battle for sexual integrity, you must let
go of past emotional pain. Maybe a father who was absent, either
emotionally or physically, wounded you. Maybe the distance in
your relationship with your mother left you feeling desperately
lonely. Perhaps your siblings or friends never treated you with dignity
or respect. If you were abused in any way (physically, sexually, or verbally) as a child, maybe you have anger and pain that has yet to be
reconciled.

Perhaps old lovers took advantage of your vulnerabilities, strung you
along, or were unfaithful to you. Or maybe you've never understood
why God allowed —— to happen (you fill in the blank). Regardless
of its source, we must surrender the pain from our past in order to
stand strong in the battle for sexual and emotional integrity. 📖

Use the chart on the next page to process some of the past emotional pain you have
experienced that has possibly left you vulnerable to sexual and/or emotional compromise. If you have more than one relationship to reconcile in this way, you may
reproduce this chart.

🐗 HARVESTING FULFILLMENT
(Applying the Truth)

📖 Why is [fear] such a hindrance? Because *fear* is the opposite of faith.… How can we focus on what we know God will do when we think we are doomed? Such lack of faith says to God, "Even though

Who is the person who caused my past emotional pain? How?	
How did this make me feel?	
How did this event/relationship make me vulnerable to temptation?	
How does this still affect me?	
What personal pain may have caused this person to hurt me?	
How does my unforgiveness affect this person?	
How does my unforgiveness affect me and my loved ones?	
How would my forgiveness affect this person?	
How would my forgiveness affect me and my loved ones?	
Can I cancel this debt as Jesus canceled mine? Why or why not?	
How can I pray for this person?	
How can I avoid causing this same pain in others' lives?	

you've carried me this far, you are probably going to fail me now, aren't you?"...

The same is true in our battle against sexual and emotional compromise. Many women are steeped in the fear of being alone, the fear of not being taken care of, the fear of not having another man on the hook in case the current one gets away. We can be so afraid of compromising tomorrow that we fail to take notice and celebrate the fact that we are standing firm today. 📖

4. Is it easier for you to imagine intimacy in a new relationship than to cultivate intimacy in the relationship you already have with your husband or with God? Why or why not?

5. Why do you think some women fear genuine intimacy (such as revealing our innermost thoughts to our husbands or to God), yet crave superficial intimacy (such as a rendezvous with an attractive stranger)?

6. How can we cultivate the courage to engage fully in genuine intimacy with our husbands and with God rather than seeking escape routes (fantasy, emotional affairs, and so on)?

❧ GROWING TOGETHER
(Sharing the Truth in Small-Group Discussion)

📖 One day as I was beating myself up for yet another emotional affair, my best friend interrupted me with these sobering words: "Do you know what you are saying about the blood that Jesus shed for you when you refuse to forgive yourself for your past? You are saying that His blood wasn't good enough for you. It didn't have enough power to cleanse you." She was right. Underlying all of my self-pity was the belief that what Jesus did for me couldn't possibly be enough to rid me of my stain. I needed some special miracle to set me free, and until I got that miracle, I had to beat myself up as an act of penance. 📖

7. Why do you think it is much harder to forgive ourselves for mistakes in judgment than to forgive others?

8. What do you think God would say to the woman who can't seem to forgive herself? Do you know someone (including yourself) who needs to hear this message? How can you relay His feelings to her?

9. Of the three issues discussed in this chapter (past emotional pain, present pride, and future fear), which issue(s) did you recognize that you need to personally surrender? Why?

10. What victory is gained as a result of this surrender? How will you be affected by this victory? How does that make you feel and why?

*L*ord, thank You for showing us that the way to victory
is through surrendering our past emotional pain, our present
prideful sins, and our future fear. Help us to let go of the things
that hinder our spiritual growth and make us vulnerable to temptation. Free us to enjoy the sexual and emotional fulfillment that
You desire for us to experience. In the name of Jesus. Amen.

rebuilding bridges

Read chapter 10 in *Every Woman's Battle*.

🍃 PLANTING GOOD SEEDS
(Personally Seeking God's Truth)

As you seek to cultivate a greater level of genuine intimacy in your marriage, some good seeds to plant in your heart include:

> For this reason a man will leave his father and mother and be united to his wife, and they will become one flesh. The man and his wife were both naked, and they felt no shame.
> (Genesis 2:24-25)

> My command is this: Love each other as I have loved you. Greater love has no one than this, that [she] lay down [her] life for [her] friends. (John 15:12-13)

1. Is your husband your closest, most intimate friend? If not, how specifically can you cultivate this kind of friendship? How would this benefit you? your marriage?

As you consider any walls that separate you and your husband's feelings for one another, a good seed to plant in your heart is James 5:16:

> Therefore confess your sins to each other and pray for each other so that you may be healed.

2. If confession is so good for an individual's soul, what effect can it have on a couple? Why?

✎ WEEDING OUT DECEPTION
(Recognizing the Truth)

> 📖 Imagine wanting to give a squirrel a nut. How would you do it? Would you chase the squirrel around the yard, grab him by his scrawny neck, and force the nut into his chubby cheeks? Of course not. You cannot require a squirrel to take a nut from you. However, you can inspire the squirrel to do this by simply placing a nut in your open palm, lying down beneath a tree, and falling asleep. When it's the squirrel's idea to take the nut, he'll do it.
>
> Communicating intimately with our husbands is very similar to giving a squirrel a nut. Requiring it is futile. Intimacy can, however, be inspired. 📖

3. Have you attempted to force the issue of intimacy in your marriage? How, specifically, have you done this? Has it worked for you? Why or why not?
4. Through reading this chapter, what ideas have you gleaned for a more effective approach to cultivating intimacy?

> 📖 Discovering a new level of intimacy in your marriage may be very difficult if you can't let your husband see completely into you. As I mentioned previously, intimacy can best be understood by breaking

the word down into syllables: *in-to-me-see.* Marital secrets serve no purpose but to alienate you from the only one who can provide the level of intimacy you truly desire as a sexual being. If you keep secrets from each other, you may build a wall between you and ultimate sexual and emotional fulfillment.

However, through humble confession and eventual restoration of trust, you can turn those walls into bridges that will bring the two of you closer together than ever before. 📖

5. Have secrets formed a wall between you and ultimate fulfillment in your marriage relationship? If your husband could see into your mind and heart, would he find any surprises or bitter disappointments there? Why or why not?

6. If harboring a secret causes you to live in fear of your husband's knowing the truth, what effect does that have on you and your relationship? What do you fear most about being honest? Why?

7. If this fear became a reality, would it be any worse than living the rest of your life harboring secrets and undermining genuine intimacy in your marriage? Is the fulfillment you stand to gain worth the risk of being honest and letting him see into your heart and mind? Why or why not?

8. If your husband were to reveal all of the good, the bad, and the ugly in his heart and mind in an effort to cultivate genuine intimacy and accountability in your relationship, could you grant him the same grace that God grants to you? Is your love and commitment unconditional? Why or why not?

🐛 HARVESTING FULFILLMENT
(Applying the Truth)

📖 Genuine sexual intimacy involves all components of our sexuality—the physical, mental, emotional, and spiritual. When these four are combined, the result is an elixir that stirs the soul, heals the heart, boggles the mind, and genuinely satisfies. 📖

📖 Once a woman experiences the intimacy of being mentally, emotionally, and spiritually naked before her husband and feeling as if she is loved for who she truly is on the inside, her natural response will be to want to give the outside package physically to her admirer. Notice I said *want to,* not *feel that she has to.* Our desire to give our bodies as a trophy to the man who has captivated our hearts and committed his faithfulness to us sets the stage for genuine sexual fulfillment. Sex performed merely out of obligation or duty will never satisfy you (or him) like presenting your passion-filled mind, body, heart, and soul to your husband on a silver platter, inviting your lover to come into your garden and taste its choice fruits (see Song of Songs 4:16). 📖

📖 God designed sex to be shared between two bodies, two minds, two hearts, and two spirits which unite together to become a one-flesh union. If you've never experienced this one-flesh union in your marriage, then you are missing out on one of the most earth-shattering and fulfilling moments of your life!

So how can you move from having "just sex" to experiencing a form of lovemaking that satisfies every fiber of your being? By understanding that sex is actually a form of worshiping God that a husband and wife enter into together. When two become one flesh physically, mentally, emotionally, and spiritually, they are saying to God, "Your plan for our sexual and emotional fulfillment is a good plan. We choose your plan instead of our own." 📖

9. Does reading these passages make you wonder if you have missed something in your sex life with your husband? If so, can you identify what specifically happens in the bedroom (either inside your mind or between the two of you) that hinders such sexual intimacy? How can that be overcome?

10. What would it take for you to *want* to give your mind, body, heart, and soul to your husband on a silver platter? Write your answer as a prayer to God.

🍂 GROWING TOGETHER
(Sharing the Truth in Small-Group Discussion)

Read through the "Intimacy Busters and Intimacy Boosters" chart at the close of chapter 10 on page 159. Then answer the following questions in a group or in smaller groups:

11. Which intimacy busters have you struggled with in the past?
12. How have you overcome those issues, and what advice do you have for other women currently struggling in those areas?
13. Which intimacy boosters have you discovered to be helpful? What effect have they had on your ultimate fulfillment? on your marriage relationship?
14. What intimacy busters could you add to this list? How do they affect couples? How can they be overcome?
15. What intimacy boosters might you add to this list? How can a woman implement those into her relationship? What benefits might result?

Father God, thank You for the incredible gift of sexual intimacy within marriage. We invite You to sanctify our bedrooms and help us enjoy being one flesh with our husbands. Help us to recognize walls that divide us and teach us how to turn those into bridges that reunite us. We ask this in Your Son's name. Amen.

retreating with the Lord

Read chapter 11 in *Every Woman's Battle*.

🪴 PLANTING GOOD SEEDS
(Personally Seeking God's Truth)

As you cultivate a more intimate friendship with God, plant Proverbs 22:11 in your heart:

> [She] who loves a pure heart and whose speech is gracious
> will have the king for [her] friend.

1. On a scale of 1 to 10, how intimate do you feel your friendship with the Lord is? What would be required to increase that number?

As you consider the awesome privilege of being a child of the King, a good seed to plant in your heart is Galatians 4:4-6:

> God sent his Son, born of a woman, born under law, to redeem those
> under law, that we might receive the full rights of [daughters]. Because
> you are [daughters], God sent the Spirit of his Son into our hearts, the
> Spirit who calls out, "Abba, Father."

2. What does this verse mean to you? Why?

As you seek to embrace the magnitude of God's faithfulness, righteousness, and lavish love for you, some good seeds to plant in your heart are:

> I am my beloved's and my beloved is mine. (Song of
> Solomon 6:3, RSV)

> I will betroth you to me forever; I will betroth you in righteousness
> and justice, in love and compassion. I will betroth you in faithful-
> ness, and you will acknowledge the LORD. (Hosea 2:19-20)

> Your love, O LORD, reaches to the heavens,
>   your faithfulness to the skies.
> Your righteousness is like the mighty mountains,
>   your justice like the great deep....
>   How priceless is your unfailing love!
> Both high and low among [women]
>   find refuge in the shadow of your wings.
> They feast on the abundance of your house;
>   you give them drink from your river of delights. (Psalm 36:5-8)

3. Do you feel as if you are feasting on the abundance of God's house and drinking from His river of delights, or are you starving spiritually, wondering why
   you are unfulfilled in your relationships? Explain why you feel the way you do.

WEEDING OUT DECEPTION
(Recognizing the Truth)

> The groom stood alone over in the corner of the room with his
> head down. As he stared at his ring, twisting the gold band that had

just been placed on his finger by his bride, tears trickled down his
cheeks and onto his hands. That is when I noticed the nail scars.
The groom was Jesus.

He waited, but the bride never once turned her face toward her
groom. She never held His hand. She never introduced the guests
to Him. She operated independently of Him.

I awoke from my dream with a sick feeling in my stomach.
"Lord, is this how I made you feel when I was looking for love in
all the wrong places?" I wept at the thought of hurting Him so
deeply.

Unfortunately, this dream illustrates exactly what is happening
between God and millions of His people. He betroths Himself to us,
we take His name (as "Christians"), and then we go about our lives
looking for love, attention, and affection from every source under
the sun except from the Son of God, the Lover of our souls. 📖

4. In what ways do you identify with my dream above? Why?

5. Where do you look for love, attention, and affection? How successful have
   you been in finding ultimate fulfillment from these sources? What does God
   offer that other sources cannot?

🦬 HARVESTING FULFILLMENT
(Applying the Truth)

6. Of the following levels of intimacy with God discussed in this chapter, what is
   the most intimate level of relationship you've experienced with Him? What
   level are you currently experiencing and why?

   • Potter / Clay Relationship
   • Shepherd / Sheep Relationship
   • Master / Servant Relationship

- Friend / Friend Relationship
- Father / Daughter Relationship
- Groom / Bride Relationship

7. If you are not currently at the level of relationship that you desire to be with God, what ideas from this chapter can you incorporate into your life in order to cultivate such intimacy? Are there others that you can add to this list?

___ a date night with Jesus
___ walking and talking with the Lord
___ a restful rendezvous with God
___ retreating with the Lord
___ other _____
___ other _____

8. If an actual retreat sounds inviting to you, circle the idea(s) that appeal to you most:

"Past, Present, and Future" Retreat—releasing past wounds through letters of forgiveness, examining present priorities, and evaluating future spiritual, relational, professional, financial, or physical goals.

Hobby Retreat—doing what you enjoy doing most (painting, reading, writing, and so on) while enjoying time alone with the Lord.

"Prayer, Praise, and Pampering" Retreat—giving yourself a spiritual spa treatment in preparation to enter His throne room in worship.

Intercessor's Retreat—praying for those God has laid on your heart and writing notes of encouragement.

"Thanks for the Memories" Retreat—updating your photo albums and giving thanks for all of the special friends and family who adorn the pages.

"Leaving a Legacy of Love" Retreat—reflecting on the spiritual markers of your life and communicating those in a special letter to your children.

9. Do you have other ideas for retreating with the Lord or specific ways you could honor Him with extended time? If so, what are they?

10. What are your biggest hindrances to pursuing extended time alone with God? How can those be overcome?

11. Specifically, what have you to gain from pursuing such experiences with Jesus? How will doing so bring victory in the battle for sexual and emotional fulfillment?

❧ GROWING TOGETHER
(Sharing the Truth in Small-Group Discussion)

12. What in this chapter has been helpful to you, and how has it affected your thinking about intimacy with God?

> 📖 Response time is a vital part of my prayer life. He already knows what is on my heart without my saying a word. I need to make time to listen to what is on His heart because without listening I'll never have a clue. 📖

13. What percentage of your prayer time is spent talking to God, and what percentage is spent listening? If the same percentages were applied to an earthly friendship, what would the result be? Would there be mutual intimacy, or would the relationship feel one-sided?

14. Do you have a specific place, time of day, or activity that you engage in where you feel especially connected to God? If so, share that with the group.

15. If God spoke to you (or the entire group) right now, what do you think He would say? How would He say it? How would you respond?

> 📖 Anticipate [your retreat with the Lord] as an exciting date. You are running away with your Lover, not confining yourself to a convent. Be creative and bask in the beauty of intimate time alone with God.

However, let me warn you: *Experiencing this incredible pleasure can be very addictive.* My annual retreats have turned into far more frequent excursions. No human can meet our deepest needs like God can, nor should anyone be expected to. My husband doesn't mind granting me this time away because I come back revived, with a renewed sense of joy over being a bride of Christ and a fresh passion for being the wife and mother God has called me to be. I can think of no better way to spend my time. 📖

16. What are your deepest needs that no human can completely satisfy? Do you believe that God is capable of providing such satisfaction? If so, how can you allow Him to do so?

17. Write down a personal invitation to Jesus Christ, expressing your desire for Him to rendezvous with you on your next "date" or retreat. When will it be? Where? What would you like Him to do for you there?

18. What do you think Jesus' response will be? How does His response make you feel?

∞

*L*ord *Jesus, we want our relationship with You to grow and blossom into everything You desire it to be. Help us to embrace our role as Your intimate friend, Your precious child, and Your chosen bride. Draw us into Your presence each day and fill us to overflowing with Your lavish love. In Your most holy name we pray. Amen.*

all quiet on the home front

Read chapter 12 in *Every Woman's Battle*.

🪣 PLANTING GOOD SEEDS
(Personally Seeking God's Truth)

As you seek to cultivate the peace, hope and joy that comes from sexual and emotional integrity, a good seed to plant in your heart is Romans 15:13:

> May the God of hope fill you with all joy and peace as you trust in
> him, so that you may overflow with hope by the power of the Holy
> Spirit.

1. What do you need to trust God with so that you can experience joy and
   peace? How would trusting God with this part of your life give you hope?

As you pursue sexual fulfillment, plant Matthew 6:33 in your heart:

> Seek first his kingdom and his righteousness, and all these things
> will be given to you as well.

2. What does this verse mean to you? In what ways do you seek God first in your life?

3. Does your time or your life need to be rearranged so that you are seeking His kingdom and righteousness above all else? If so, how?

As you seek to overcome sexual and emotional compromise, a good seed to plant in your heart is this:

> To [her] who overcomes, I will give the right to sit with me on my throne, just as I overcame and sat down with my Father on his throne. (Revelation 3:21)

4. Looking beyond this life and into eternity, describe what you believe it will be like to sit as an overcomer with Jesus Christ on His throne. How does imagining this picture inspire you to continue pursuing sexual and emotional integrity? What can you do to ensure that you finish strong in this race toward righteousness?

⬦ WEEDING OUT DECEPTION
(Recognizing the Truth)

> 📖 I never realized how intense and chaotic my life was until I experienced the peace of living with sexual and emotional integrity. For years I had walked blindly into compromising situations, begged over dinner tables for morsels of affection, and found myself sleeping with the enemy time and time again. I consistently mistook intensity for intimacy and the concept of a peaceful relationship seemed unfathomable. 📖

5. As a result of reading this book, what things in your past do you recognize as being detrimental to your integrity and peace of mind? What effect were these issues having on you and your relationships?

6. How has your life become more peaceful as a result of avoiding such compromise? In what ways have you been strengthened as you pursue sexual integrity?

> 📖 I sat in a chair across from an imaginary "Shannon at fifteen" (the young girl I once was who was about to make all the sexual mistakes that I had just lived through). With my counselor's guidance, I was able to voice my new understanding of the pain and loneliness this fifteen-year-old had felt, sympathize with her naiveté and confusion about her sexual and emotional desires, and forgive her for the bad choices she was making and the pain that her poor judgment would cause me and many others. 📖

7. What do you know now that you wish you had known in your past relationships with men? What would you say to yourself if you could go back in time and speak face to face with that young woman?

🦃 HARVESTING FULFILLMENT
(Applying the Truth)

> 📖 I realize now that Craig was just as hurt over what I was thinking in my mind while we were having sex as I would have been if he had wanted to look at pornography while making love to me. Understanding how we each struggle to maintain sexual integrity has transformed our marriage, our bedroom in particular....
>
> I did what you recommended.... We leave on a dim light and I open my eyes anytime I sense my mind wandering outside of our bedroom. It takes concentration, but when I relax and focus completely on Craig during sex and what we are experiencing together, I feel so close to him and so much closer to God as a result! I actually enjoy sex now rather than just tolerate it and let my mind wander. I never knew it could be this deeply gratifying. 📖

8. How has your deeper understanding of men and women's unique struggles with sexual integrity affected your relationship with your husband or the men you date?

9. Do you feel that you are (or will be) able to take off your mask and share your private sexual struggles with your marriage partner? Why or why not?

10. Does this level of openness and honesty with your husband make you feel any closer to God? If so, write your own prayer of thanksgiving. If not, write a prayer asking God to help you identify and remove any barriers that may still remain between you and Him.

❧ GROWING TOGETHER
(Sharing the Truth in Small-Group Discussion)

11. What (or who) encouraged you to read *Every Woman's Battle* and go through this workbook? What were you hoping to find in its pages? What were your expectations, and were they fulfilled?

12. What did you discover in this study that you weren't expecting? How have these discoveries changed your life? your marriage? your relationships with the women in your discussion group?

> 📖 You will be tempted to resort to your old fantasies, your old masturbation habit, or your dysfunctional relational patterns. That doesn't mean that you can't have victory time and time again, however. With each thought taken captive, each inappropriate word not spoken, each extramarital advance you spurn, and each intimate sexual experience you enjoy with your husband, you will be reinforcing your victory and embracing God's plan for your sexual and emotional fulfillment. 📖

13. How will you know the difference between experiencing temptations and crossing the line in the future?

14. How can you ensure victory even though this battle will continue as long as your are living and breathing?

📖 To someone who knew the taste of defeat all too well, the thrill of victory is truly something to be savored. 📖

15. Have you experienced the taste of defeat? Describe how it tastes.
16. Have you experienced the thrill of victory? Describe how it feels.
17. Do you know anyone with the taste of defeat on her tongue? If so, how can you share with her what victory tastes like and whet her appetite for God's plan for sexual and emotional integrity? Will you commit to pray for her and for God to use you to help bring victory into her life?

∞

Lord, thank You that Your plan for my sexual and emotional fulfillment is a perfect one. Continue revealing it to me and reminding me of it, especially when my determination to walk in integrity weakens. Strengthen me in times of temptation and give me a heart that recognizes and rejoices each time Your Holy Spirit guides me toward righteousness. Continue to cultivate genuine sexual intimacy between me and my husband and draw me into a deeper, more passionate love relationship with You day by day. Thank You for Your granting me peace, hope, and joy and teaching me how to be an overcomer. I look so forward to sitting next to You on Your throne for all eternity. In Jesus' most precious and holy name. Amen.

don't keep it to yourself

Congratulations on finishing this workbook! You are well on your way to winning the battle for sexual and emotional integrity. I pray that you have learned how to guard not just your body, but your mind, heart, and mouth from sexual compromise. I pray you have discovered God's plan for ultimate sexual fulfillment and that, if you are married, you are cultivating a deeper level of intimacy with your husband than you ever imagined possible. But most of all, I hope you have tasted and seen that, in fact, the Lord is good and His plans are perfect.

If you've just completed the *Every Woman's Battle Workbook* on your own and benefited from it, let me encourage you to consider inviting a group of other women together and leading them toward discovering God's plan for sexual and emotional fulfillment as well. This can help keep you accountable, but it will also enable you to encourage and help other women who are in the battle with you. If as women we can encourage each other to open up about our struggles in this area, we will be able to get the support and help we need.

You'll find more information about starting such a group on pages 194–95 in the section titled "Questions You May Have About This Workbook."

Chapter 1

1. While this book attempts to cover the most common sexual and emotional issues affecting women, some issues that hinder fulfillment and relational satisfaction may be beyond the scope of this book.

Chapter 3

1. Stephen Arterburn, *Addicted to Love* (Ann Arbor, Mich.: Servant, 1996), 122.
2. Tim Clinton, from a class titled "Counselor Professional Identity, Function and Ethics Videotape Course," External Degree Program, Liberty University, Lynchburg, Va. Used with permission.
3. Stephen Arterburn and Fred Stoeker, *Every Man's Battle* (Colorado Springs: WaterBrook, 2000), 31.

Chapter 4

1. *The New Standard Encyclopedia*, s.v. "burlesque."
2. Chart prepared by Jack Hill to encapsulate the points made in Craig W. Ellison, "From Eden to the Couch," *Christian Counseling Today* 10, no. 1, 2002, 30. Used with permission.
3. Kari Torjesen Malcom, *Women at the Crossroads* (Downers Grove, Ill.: InterVarsity, 1982), 78-9.
4. *Glamour,* October 2002.
5. *Redbook,* October 2002.
6. *Cosmopolitan,* September 2002.
7. Diane Passno, *Feminism: Mystique or Mistake?* (Wheaton, Ill.: Tyndale, 2000), 7-8, 20-1.

8. Carle Zimmerman, *Family and Civilization* (New York: Harper and Brothers, 1947), 776-7.

9. Tim Clinton, from a class titled "Counselor Professional Identity, Function and Ethics Videotape Course," External Degree Program, Liberty University, Lynchburg, Va. Used with permission.

10. Neil T. Anderson, *Living Free in Christ* (Ventura, Calif.: Regal, 1993), 278. Used with permission.

Chapter 5

1. Adapted from Linda Dillow and Lorraine Pintus, *Intimate Issues* (Colorado Springs: WaterBrook, 1999), 199-201.

2. Dillow and Pintus, *Intimate Issues,* 203-4.

Chapter 6

1. Stephen Arterburn, *Addicted to Love* (Ann Arbor, Mich.: Servant, 1996), 46.

Chapter 8

1. American Social Health Association, *Sexually Transmitted Diseases in America: How Many Cases and at What Cost?* (Menlo Park, Calif.: Kaiser Family Foundation, 1998), 5.

2. Steve Marshall, "Elderly AIDS," *USA Today,* 7 July 1994, 3A.

3. No author given, *HPV Press Release,* Medical Institute for Sexual Health (MISH), Austin, Tex., 9 May 2000.

4. Susan C. Weller, "A Meta-Analysis of Condom Effectiveness in Reducing Sexually Transmitted HIV," *UTMB News,* University of Texas Medical Branch—Galveston, 7 June 1993, Social Science and Medicine, 36:36:1635-44.

Chapter 9

1. Ellen Michaud, "Discover the Power of Forgiveness." *Prevention* 51, no. 1, January 1999, 110-5, 163-4.

2. These steps are explained in more detail in the *Every Woman's Battle Workbook*.

Chapter 10

1. Mike Mason, *The Mystery of Marriage* (Portland, Oreg.: Multnomah, 1985), 121.
2. Stephen Arterburn and Fred Stoeker, *Every Man's Battle* (Colorado Springs: WaterBrook, 2000), 138.

Chapter 12

1. Share the secrets to discovering God's plan for sexual and emotional fulfillment by starting a group in your church or circle of friends to journey through the *Every Woman's Battle Workbook* together.

about the author

Shannon Ethridge is the best-selling author of *Every Woman's Battle* and co-author of the award-winning *Every Young Woman's Battle,* both of which have remained on the bestseller list since their release and been reprinted in seven different languages.

She's written ten other books, including *Preparing Your Daughter for Every Woman's Battle* and *Every Woman's Marriage.*

Previously a youth pastor and abstinence educator, Shannon has a master's degree in counseling and human relations from Liberty University, and she speaks regularly on the Teen Mania Ministries campus and in a variety of other church and college settings.

She lives in East Texas with her husband, Greg, and their two children, Erin and Matthew.

Visit her Web site at www.shannonethridge.com.

Win the War on
Sexual Temptation at Every Age

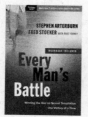 *Every Man's Battle: Winning the War on Sexual Temptation One Victory at a Time*
By Stephen Arterburn and Fred Stoeker
with Mike Yorkey
ISBN 978-0-307-45797-4
Ideal for ages: 18+

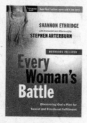 *Every Woman's Battle: Discovering God's Plan for Sexual and Emotional Fulfillment*
By Shannon Ethridge
with foreword and afterword by Stephen Arterburn
ISBN 978-0-307-45798-1
Ideal for ages: 18+

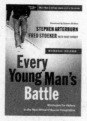 *Every Young Man's Battle: Strategies for Victory in the Real World of Sexual Temptation*
By Stephen Arterburn and Fred Stoeker
with Mike Yorkey
ISBN 978-0-307-45799-8
Ideal for ages: 12-17

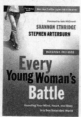 *Every Young Woman's Battle: Guarding Your Mind, Heart, and Body in a Sex-Saturated World*
By Shannon Ethridge and Stephen Arterburn
with foreword by Josh McDowell
ISBN 978-0-307-45800-1
Ideal for ages: 12-17